how to feed your baby
with healthy homemade meals

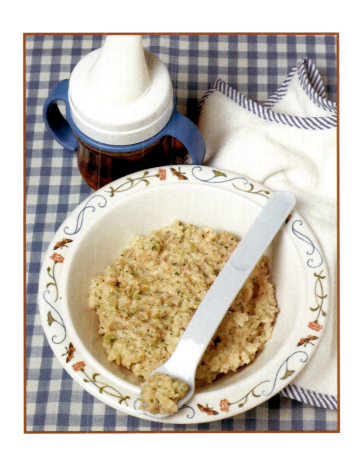

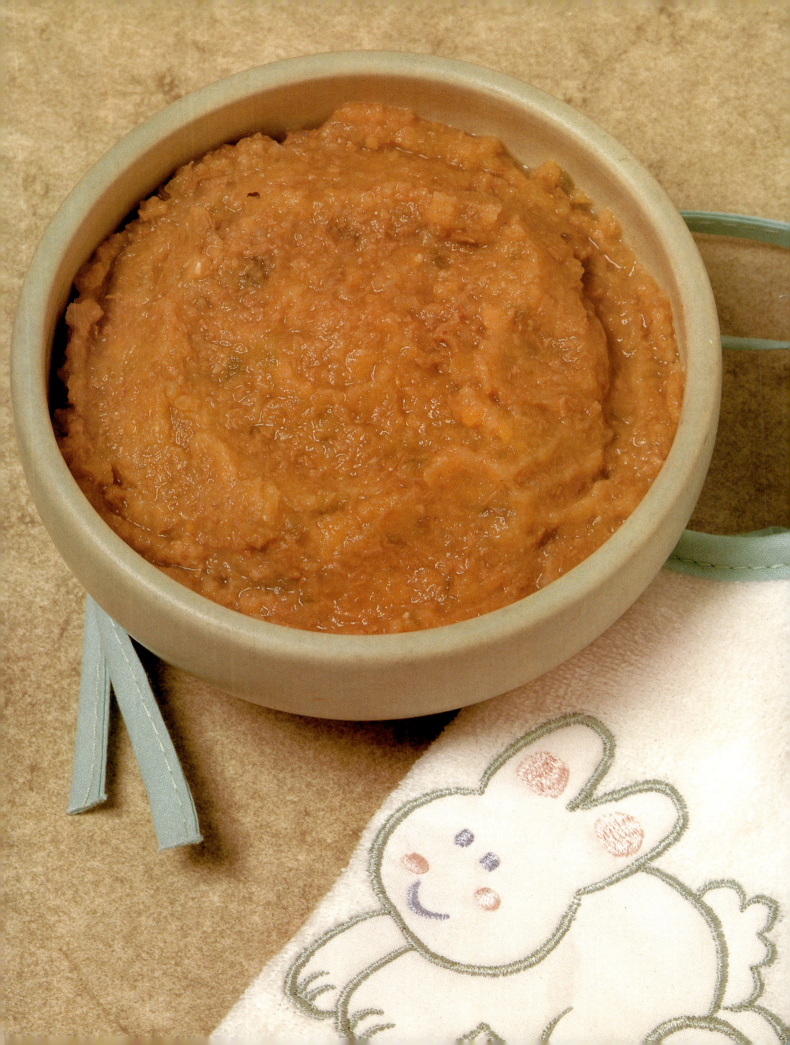

how to feed your baby
with healthy homemade meals

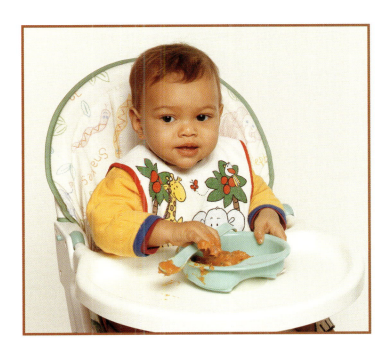

Give your baby the very best start in life
with 50 easy-to-make step-by-step tempting
recipes for deliciously wholesome purées
and nutritional first solids

Sara Lewis

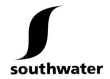

southwater

Dedication: To my children, William aged 1 who has eaten every recipe in the book with great enthusiasm and Alice, aged 5, the fussiest of fussy eaters.

This edition is published by Southwater, an imprint of Anness Publishing Ltd, Hermes House, 88–89 Blackfriars Road, London SE1 8HA
tel. 020 7401 2077; fax 020 7633 9499

www.southwaterbooks.com; www.annesspublishing.com

If you like the images in this book and would like to investigate using them for publishing, promotions or advertising, please visit our website
www.practicalpictures.com for more information.

UK agent: The Manning Partnership Ltd; tel. 01225 478444; fax 01225 478440; sales@manning-partnership.co.uk
UK distributor: Grantham Book Services Ltd; tel. 01476 541080; fax 01476 541061; orders@gbs.tbs-ltd.co.uk
North American agent/distributor: National Book Network; tel. 301 459 3366; fax 301 429 5746; www.nbnbooks.com
Australian agent/distributor: Pan Macmillan Australia; tel. 1300 135 113; fax 1300 135 103; customer.service@macmillan.com.au
New Zealand agent/distributor: David Bateman Ltd; tel. (09) 415 7664; fax (09) 415 8892

ETHICAL TRADING POLICY

At Anness Publishing we believe that business should be conducted in an ethical and ecologically sustainable way, with respect for the environment and a proper regard to the replacement of the natural resources we employ.

As a publisher, we use a lot of wood pulp to make high-quality paper for printing, and that wood commonly comes from spruce trees. We are therefore currently growing more than 500,000 trees in two Scottish forest plantations near Aberdeen – Berrymoss (130 hectares/320 acres) and West Touxhill (125 hectares/305 acres). The forests we manage contain twice the number of trees employed each year in paper-making for our books.

Because of this ongoing ecological investment programme, you, as our customer, can have the pleasure and reassurance of knowing that a tree is being cultivated on your behalf to naturally replace the materials used to make the book you are holding.

Our forestry programme is run in accordance with the UK Woodland Assurance Scheme (UKWAS) and will be certified by the internationally recognized Forest Stewardship Council (FSC). The FSC is a non-government organization dedicated to promoting responsible management of the world's forests. Certification ensures forests are managed in an environmentally sustainable and socially responsible way. For further information about this scheme, go to www.annesspublishing.com/trees

Publisher: Joanna Lorenz
Editorial Director: Judith Simons
Editors: Emma Wish and Molly Perham
Designer: Sue Storey
Special Photography: John Freeman
Stylist: Judy Williams
Home Economists: Sara Lewis, Jacqueline Clarke
and Petra Jackson

© Anness Publishing Ltd 1996, updated 2006

A CIP catalogue record for this book is available from the British Library.

Previously published as *Happy Healthy Baby Cookbook*

ACKNOWLEDGEMENTS

• I am particularly grateful to the Department of Health for reading and approving the section on food for babies.
• National Dairy Council Nutrition Service
• Healthy Education Authority
• Dr Nigel Dickie from Heinz Baby Foods
• The British Dietetic Association
• The Health Visitors Association
• For Broadstone Communications for their invaluable help supplying Kenward equipment for recipe testing and photography
• Hand-painted china plates, bowls and mugs from Cosmo Place Studio
• Tupperware for plain-coloured plastic bowls, plates, feeder beakers and cups
• Cole and Mason for children's ware
• Royal Doulton for Bunnykins china
• Spode for blue and white Edwardian Childhood china.

PICTURE CREDITS

Bubbles: pages 85br (Jacqui Farrow); pages 25t, 39, 65tr (Lois Joy Thurston); page 29t (F Rombout); page 73 (S Price); pages 83t, 84t (Ian West).
Lupe Cunha: pages 30, 36/37, 42, 45t, 56, 75.
Greg Evans: page 78.
Sally and Richard Greenhill: page 62t.
Lyons Waddell: page 59t.
Reflections/Jennie Woodcock: pages 63b, 64tr, 74/75, 77, 85cr, 87.

NOTES

• For all recipes, quantities are given in both metric and imperial measures and, where appropriate, measures are also given in standard cups and spoons. Follow one set, but not a mixture, because they are not interchangeable.
• Standard spoon and cup measures are level.
1 tsp = 5ml, 1 tbsp = 15ml, 1 cup = 250ml/8fl oz
• Australian tablespoons are 20ml. Australian readers should use 3 tsp in place of 1 tbsp for measuring small quantities.
• American pints are 16fl oz/2 cups. American readers should use 20fl oz/2.5 cups in place of 1 pint when measuring liquids.
• Electric oven temperatures in this book are for conventional ovens. When using a fan oven, the temperature will probably need to be reduced by about 10–20°C/20–40°F. Since ovens vary, you should check with your manufacturer's instruction book for guidance.
• Use medium (US large) eggs unless otherwise stated.

CONTENTS

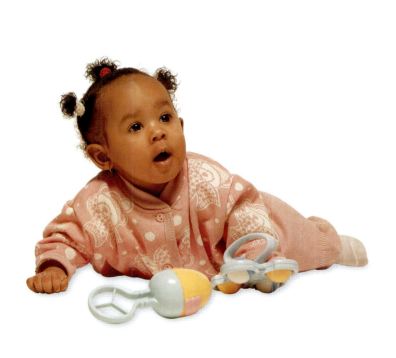
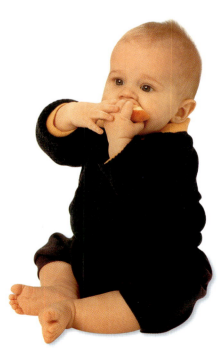

INTRODUCTION

Introducing your baby to the delights of solid food heralds the beginning of a new and exciting stage in her development. You will know she is ready when she seems unsatisfied after a milk feed, or shows an interest in what you are eating. Although it will be a few months yet before she is able to share in family meals fully, the foods that you give your baby now are important not only for their nutritional benefits but also in laying down the first foundations for a healthy diet through childhood and beyond.

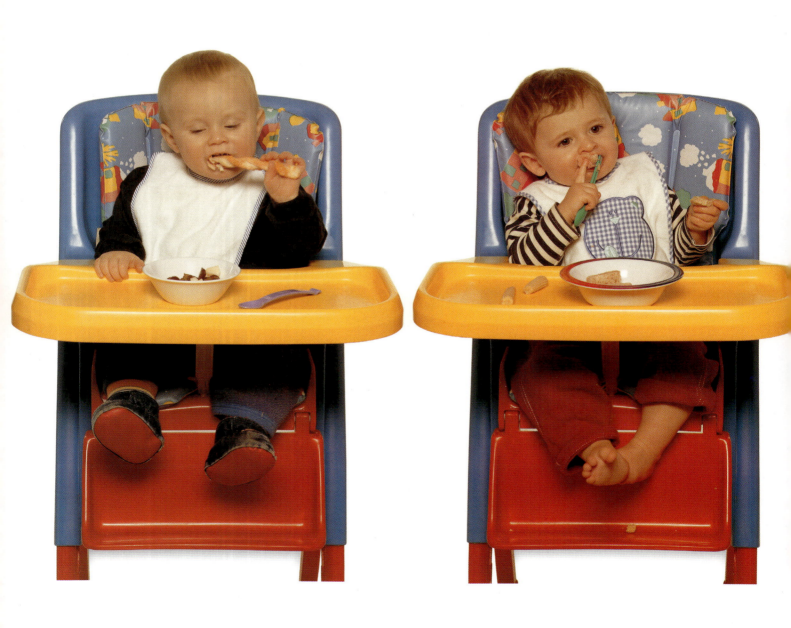

There are several important factors to consider when planning your baby's diet: at what stage to begin weaning; what foods to serve and when; and how to prepare foods quickly and easily while still providing the nutrient-dense diet babies need. Your baby's progression from milk feeds to solids will be gradual. Start with baby rice that is barely warm and only slightly thicker than milk, before moving on to those first few spoonfuls of puréed vegetables and fruits. Then, stage by stage, you will be able to introduce your baby to a tempting array of new flavours and textures.

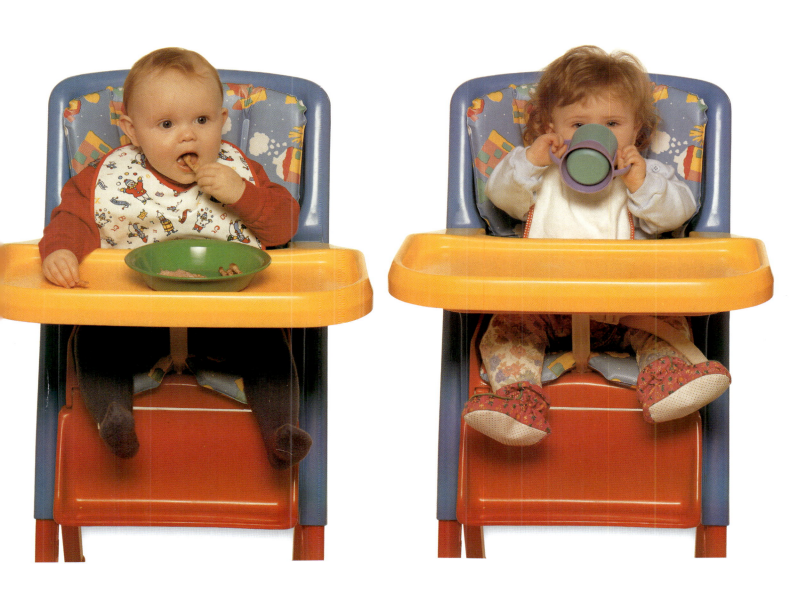

FIRST FOODS

ALTHOUGH DURING THE FIRST FEW YEARS OF ANY BABY'S LIFE, FOOD, DIET AND NUTRITION ARE VITALLY IMPORTANT TO BUILD A HEALTHY AND ENERGETIC CHILD AND TO DEVELOP GOOD EATING HABITS THAT WILL SEE THE INFANT SAFELY THROUGH CHILDHOOD, THERE IS A REAL SHORTAGE OF RELIABLE, PRACTICAL INFORMATION ON THE SUBJECT.

This book aims to outline all you need to know about feeding your baby in one volume. It is packed with over 50 recipes, all beautifully illustrated with colour pictures. Each recipe includes clear step-by-step instructions, which will ensure success every time, whether you are making your child's first purées, serving simple and tasty finger foods, or introducing those first tempting toddler dishes to your developing child.

In the very early days, all a baby needs is milk, but as it grows so too will its nutritional needs. By six months most babies will have doubled their birth weight and will be ready to begin mini-mouthfuls of simple mashed food.

Although this marks an exciting time in your baby's development, it can also cause immense worry for a new parent. We all want to provide the best for our child, and what better start in life is there than to begin laying down the foundations of a healthy diet? But what do you do if your child won't eat, or just spits out those delicious spoonfuls of food that you have so lovingly prepared?

FIRST FOODS

Here is everything you need to know about introducing those first few spoonfuls of smooth mashed or puréed foods, such as when to begin weaning, the signs to look out for that show your baby is ready, which foods to serve and when, and which foods to avoid. It also includes invaluable advice on basic equipment, plus nutritional information, helpful guidelines on food preparation, and masses of colourful and exciting recipes with which to tempt your baby.

You will almost certainly find that friends, relatives, health professionals and magazines will offer you differing and sometimes contradictory advice. Some will be genuinely useful, while some will be outdated or inappropriate: the difficulty is sorting through the well-meaning confusion to find

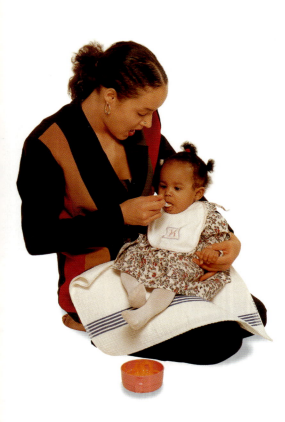

Left: You can sit your baby in your lap while feeding. Use a dish towel to protect your clothes.

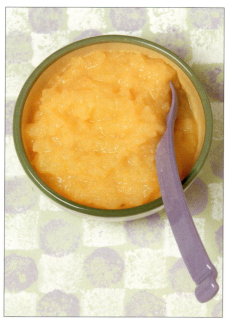

Above: *Apple and Orange Fool is just one of the many delicious recipes for your baby.*

something that is reliable. This book is based on the latest government information and advice, and aims to offer helpful advice in accordance with those guidelines

FOOD AND YOUR BABY

Childrens' nutritional needs are very different from our own. Forget about low-fat and high-fibre diets. Young children require nutrient-dense foods to meet their rapid levels of growth. Requirements for protein and energy are high in proportion to the child's size. Tiny tummies mean children are unable to eat large quantities of food, while at the same time they are usually very active. Their appetites can vary

Right: *Start with simple vegetable purées when your baby is around six months old.*

enormously, but the range of foods that they will eat may be very limited. Consequently, it is vital that the foods which are eaten contain a variety of nutrients, in combination with calories, while still fitting in with family meals. High-fibre foods can be very filling without providing sufficient levels of protein, vitamins and minerals.

For young infants, fat is the major source of dietary energy: both breast milk and infant formula contribute about 50 per cent of energy as fat. As your child progresses to a mixed diet, the proportion of energy supplied by fat decreases and is replaced by carbohydrate. However, it is important that the energy your baby takes in is provided by fat until she reaches the age of two because too much carbohydrate may be too bulky for a young infant.

Adequate energy is necessary to sustain growth. Fat is a very useful source of energy and the main source of the fat-soluble vitamins, A, D, E and K, while also providing essential fatty acids that the body cannot make itself. It is best to obtain fat from foods that contain other essential nutrients, such as full-fat (whole) milk, cheese, yogurt, lean meat and small quantities of oily fish.

Try to include a portion of carbohydrate in every meal once your child is over nine months: for example, bread, potatoes, rice or pasta for energy. Encourage young children to eat a variety of fruit and vegetables. As with adults, try to keep salt intakes to a minimum; fried foods or very sugary foods should be discouraged and served only as a special treat.

Obviously, having a healthy, well-balanced diet is essential for any age group, but acquiring social skills is also important. Our children learn from us,

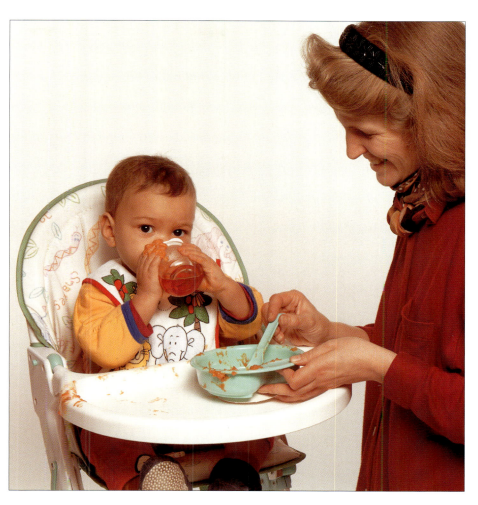

and so it is vital to eat together as a family, if not every single day, then as often as possible. It is never too early for the youngest member of the family to start learning how to behave at the table – though, to begin with, it will no doubt be a relatively messy experience. Your child will soon come to regard family meals as a sociable and enjoyable time.

As well as providing vital nutritional information and advice for your growing child, we hope that this book will help minimize any problems and make meal-times fun for your baby and the entire family.

Right: *Babies are easily encouraged to take pleasure in their food, however simple. Give your baby finger food as well as a spoon and bowl.*

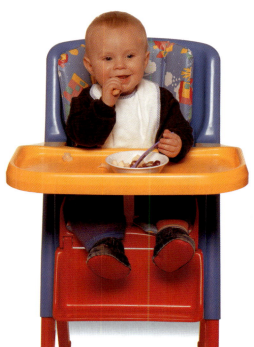

Weaning from Milk Feeds to Solids

Most babies are ready to begin those first few mini-mouthfuls of mashed or puréed foods at around six months and will soon progress to a mixed diet of solid foods. By this age, babies need the extra energy, protein, iron and other essential nutrients that are found in solids in order to help them develop and grow. Your baby will also be progressing from sucking to biting and chewing – as many breast-feeding mothers find out!

Remember that every baby has individual needs, so don't be surprised if your baby seems ready for solids a little earlier or later than other babies of the same age. Don't feel pressurized by friends with young babies, or helpful relatives. Be guided by your own baby.

Below: *Your baby will very quickly take an interest in your hand and the spoon, and will play as she eats.*

Right: *When the signs are right, start your baby with a few mouthfuls of mashed vegetables or fruit after a milk feed, or in the middle of one, if this works better. If the food is hot, make sure you stir it and test it before giving it to your baby.*

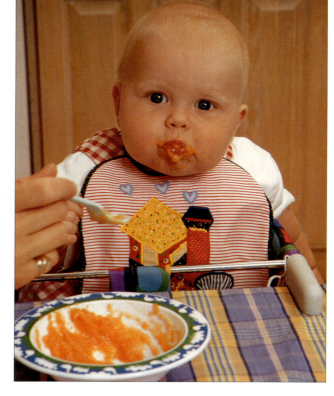

Below right: *When your baby starts picking up food and putting it into his mouth, he is ready to try solid foods.*

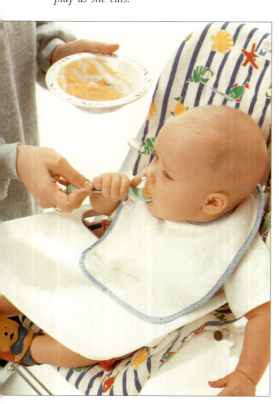

WHAT TO LOOK OUT FOR

If your baby:
- still seems hungry after you have increased the milk feed
- wants feeding more frequently
- shows a real interest in the foods that you are eating
- picks up food and puts it into mouth, wanting to chew
- can sit up

If your baby is showing some or all of these signs, then she is probably ready to begin solids. Some babies may show these signs earlier than six months, but the majority should not be given solid foods before six months as their digestive systems can't cope. Be guided as well by any family history of allergies, eczema or asthma. Studies suggest that babies fed on breast or formula milk a bit longer are less likely to develop such complaints.

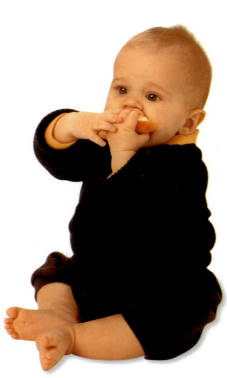

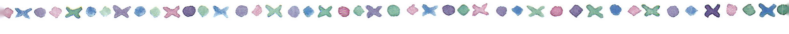

In the early days of weaning, your baby is not dependent on solid food for the supply of nutrients as this is still met by milk feeds. Don't worry if she only takes a taste of food to begin with – the actual experience of taking food off a spoon is the most important thing at this stage. However, as your baby grows older, solid foods are essential for supplying all the vital minerals and vitamins she needs.

WHAT ABOUT MILK FEEDS?
During the early stages of weaning, solids are given in addition to normal feeds of breast or formula milk. As mixed feeding continues, your baby will naturally cut down on the number of milk feeds, but milk will remain an important part of a child's diet.

Up to six months your baby should be having four to five milk feeds a day, and by age one your baby needs at least 600ml/1 pint full-fat (whole) milk a day. Milk will still contribute 40 percent of the energy she uses up. Health professionals recommend that children should not be given cow's milk as their main drink until after 12 months, due to low levels of iron and vitamins C and D. Mothers may be advised to go on to fortified formula when breast feeding has finished. Small amounts of cow's milk may be used in cooking from six months, but it is better to use formula milk.

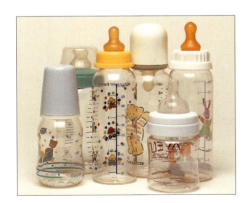

Above: *Bottles are a wonderful aid, but try to wean your baby off them by age one, or the sucking habit can be difficult to break.*

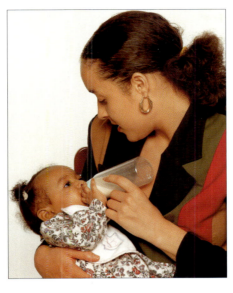

Above: *Every baby is different. There is no need to be worried if your baby seems ready for solids earlier or later than other babies.*

Full-fat cow's milk can be given to children between one and two, while semi-skimmed (low-fat) milk can be gradually introduced to those over two, providing the child eats well. Skimmed milk should not be given to children under five.

Only give pasteurized milk to children. UHT or long-life milk is a useful standby for holidays and travelling as it doesn't need to be refrigerated. However, once opened treat it as full-fat pasteurized milk.

Some people prefer to give goat's or sheep's milk believing it is less allergenic and offers additional nourishment, although this cannot be substantiated. Goat's milk is deficient in folic acid and must not be given to babies under six months. Boil goat's milk before use, as it may be sold unpasteurized.

WEANING FROM BREAST OR BOTTLE
You can go on breast feeding your baby, as well as giving solid food, for as long as you wish. However, many mothers are quite relieved when their baby is happy to try a feeder

cup or bottle along with their lunch-time "solid" meal. Once solids become established the number of daytime milk feeds naturally tails off, with just the special morning and evening comfort feeds continuing until you and your baby are ready to stop.

Whether bottle or breast and bottle feeding, try to wean your baby off the bottle completely by the age of one. Otherwise your baby may find it difficult to give the bottle up, and comfort sucking on a teat can be a hard habit to break.

Once your baby can sit up, you can introduce a lidded feeding cup, initially at one meal a day, then at two and so on. But do make sure that you cuddle your baby while giving a drink, so that the baby still enjoys the closeness and security of being with her mother or father. There may be a few setbacks when your baby is teething or unwell, but be guided by your baby.

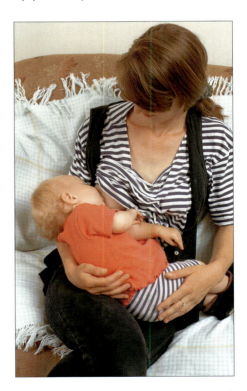

Above: *It won't all happen at once: a mixed period of feeding with breast, bottle and simple solids is perfectly natural and healthy.*

Introducing Solid Food

Many parents find that around late morning, after their baby's morning sleep, is the best time to introduce solids. The baby is happy and nicely hungry without being frantic. Offer a small milk feed to take the edge off her immediate hunger and make her feel secure, and then go on to offer solid food. Finish with the rest of the milk feed or "second side".

SITTING COMFORTABLY

If you are feeding a slightly younger baby, you might like to hold her securely on your lap while offering the first spoonfuls. However, most babies will be comfortable fed in a high-chair.

FIRST SPOONFULS

Baby rice is often the most successful first food because its milky taste and soft texture seem vaguely familiar to the baby. Begin by trying a teaspoonful of bought baby rice, add a little previously boiled water, expressed breast milk or formula milk as the pack directs, and mix to make a smooth runny purée, slightly thicker than milk. Test the temperature on the edge of your lip, it should be just lukewarm – too hot and you may put the baby off solids completely. Offer tiny amounts on the end of a sterilized teaspoon. Go at your baby's pace and don't try to hurry things.

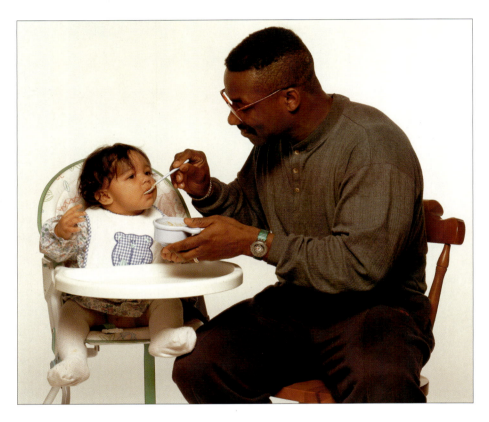

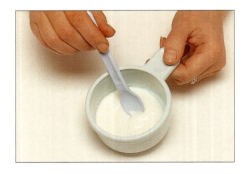

Above: *First baby rice will be barely warm, and only very slightly thicker than milk.*

Learning to eat from a spoon is quite a skill, and your baby may start spitting out the food until she has mastered the technique of taking food off the spoon and transferring it to the back of her mouth. It is possible that she may not like the taste of the food. If you started with baby rice, then go on to potato or parsnip purée mixed into the baby rice. If your baby seems reluctant, then abandon the feed and go back to breast or bottle feeding – your baby may simply not be ready for solids yet.

You could try solids again a few days later – there's plenty of time. Never force-feed and never add solid foods to a baby's bottle, as it can lead to choking, which can be dangerous.

BABY APPEARS TO GAG

Some babies just cannot cope with solids at first and may seem distressed and almost gag on the food.

Above: *At about six months your baby will be ready to sit safely in a high-chair. You should always use a strap to make sure she is safely fastened in.*

Try thinning down the food even more, as it may be too thick. Alternatively, you may be putting too much on the spoon: try offering your baby a little less. If neither of these seems to help, stop solids and breast or bottle feed as usual, giving your baby plenty of reassuring cuddles. Try again in a few days' or weeks' time.

INTRODUCING VEGETABLES

After rice, gradually introduce mashed or puréed potato, carrot, parsnip and swede (rutabaga), or puréed apple or pears. As always, be guided by your baby: this is a slow process so don't try to hurry your baby if she is not ready, or you will run the risk of discouraging her altogether.

SPOON FEEDING FOR THE FIRST TIME

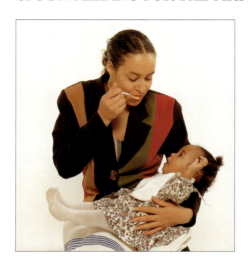 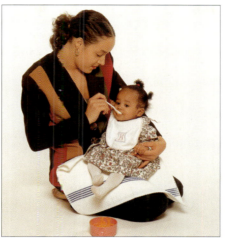 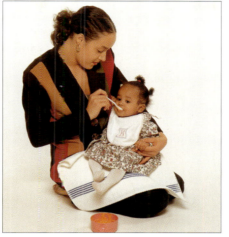

1 Sit your baby on your lap in a familiar position. Always test the temperature of the food.

2 Offer the spoon to your baby. Go slowly and if the spoon or food is rejected try again another day.

3 When your baby has taken her first solid food, sit her quietly for a little while in an upright position.

After a week or two your baby may be ready to try two mini-meals a day. Increase the amount of food to 10ml/2 tsp, even 15ml/3 tsp if your baby seems ready. You may be able to slightly reduce the amount of formula or breast milk you use to make the purée, so that it is not quite so sloppy. If your baby likes the flavour, then offer it again for a few meals before introducing a new taste. If your baby spits it out, then go back to baby rice or try mixing the new flavour with a little baby rice so that it is milder and more palatable.

Try to follow your baby's appetite and pace; most babies will stop when they have had enough. Don't be tempted to persuade your baby to finish off those last few spoonfuls. It's a bad habit to force or encourage anyone to clear the plate if they are full. If you do it with a baby, she'll probably be sick!

Adopt a feeding schedule to suit you both. In the early days it may be easier to give the baby breakfast before older children get up, or after they're at school, when the house is quieter. Six to eight weeks into solid feeding, your baby will probably be ready for three small meals a day. Again, be guided by her needs and appetite, so don't introduce a third meal until you feel she is really ready. Aim to feed your baby at roughly equal time intervals that will eventually coincide with as many family meals as possible.

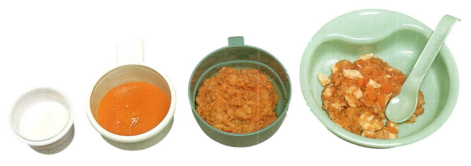

Above: *You can build up the diet from baby rice to items like mashed or puréed carrot, parsnip, apple or pear, gradually leaving more texture as your baby seems ready.*

EQUIPMENT

Choose a small plastic spoon, preferably with a shallow bowl that is gentle on your baby's gums. Look out for packs of weaning spoons in pharmacies or baby-care shops. If you don't want to buy a lot of equipment right away, you may find it useful to mix small quantities of baby rice in the sterilized cap of a bottle. Alternatively, use a small china ramekin or plastic bowl. Plastic bowls with suction feet or insulated linings are also perfectly adequate and will be useful later on when your baby gets bigger. All equipment must be scrupulously clean (and sterilized if your baby is under six-and-a-half months old).

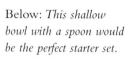

Below: *This shallow bowl with a spoon would be the perfect starter set.*

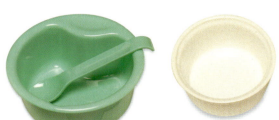

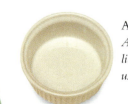

Above, left and below: *Any small dish, or even the lid of a baby's bottle, can be used for mixing and feeding.*

Below: *A bib is even more essential once your baby is taking solid foods.*

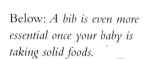

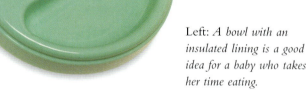

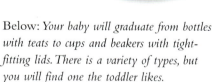

Left: *A bowl with an insulated lining is a good idea for a baby who takes her time eating.*

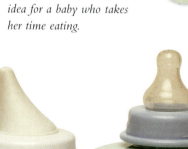

Below: *Your baby will graduate from bottles with teats to cups and beakers with tight-fitting lids. There is a variety of types, but you will find one the toddler likes.*

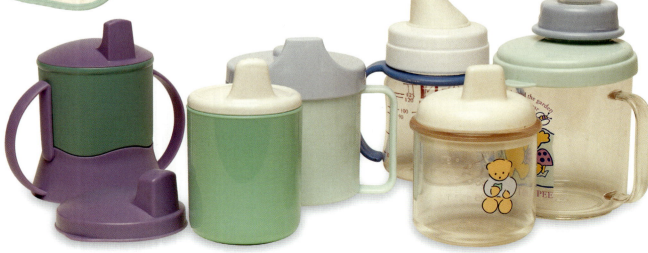

FEEDING TWINS

Probably the easiest way to feed twins is to sit the babies side by side and offer food from one bowl. Twins can get rather frustrated if you have to keep picking up different bowls and spoons. Try to be adaptable and if you find a way that works then stick with it. Encourage finger foods slightly earlier: perhaps a mini ham sandwich, cooked broccoli floret or carrot stick.

Wait until each child has finished their main course before offering dessert, as the slow eater will be distracted and want to go on to dessert too.

Looking after twins can be exhausting so you may find serving sandwiches for lunch an easier option, and this will give you a chance to eat something too. Serve cooked food for the evening meal.

DRINKS

Although your baby will need less milk for nourishment, she will still need something to drink, especially in hot weather. Always offer at least two drinks during the day and also a drink with every meal.

You can give:
- breast, formula milk or, at over one year, full-fat (whole) cow's milk
- cooled boiled water
- well-diluted pure unsweetened fruit juice

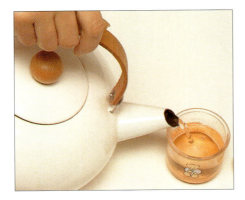

Above: *Dilute juices with boiled and cooled water.*

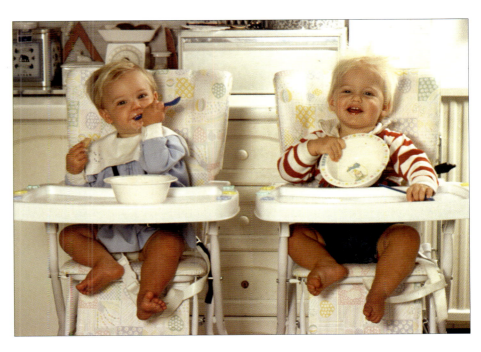

You can stop boiling the water for the baby's drinks when you stop sterilizing her feeding equipment, but always make sure you provide water from the mains supply and allow the tap to run before using it. Never use water from the hot tap.

If you have a water softener make sure that you use a tap connected directly to the mains supply and independent of the water softener. Artificially softened water is not recommended as salts are added during the softening process. Check with your doctor or health visitor before giving a baby bottled water, as the mineral content varies and you will need to choose a low-mineral brand such as those that are labelled "spring water". As a general rule, bottled water is not really necessary unless you are on holiday (vacation) where it is unsafe to drink the water.

Some fruit drinks contain a lot of added sugar, so check the label for sucrose, glucose, dextrose, fructose, maltose, syrup, honey or concentrated fruit juice. If you do give concentrated drinks to your baby, make sure you dilute them correctly, and do not give them too often. Pure fruit juices contain no

Above: *If you have twins, put their chairs side by side at meal-times.*

Below: *Drinks fill up the baby's tummy – so offer drinks after food.*

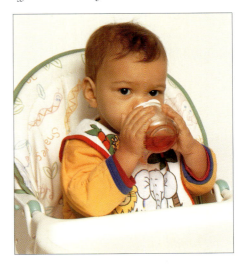

added sugar. At first, dilute them with one part juice to three parts water. The amount of water can be reduced as the child matures. Offer drinks at the end of meal times once your baby has settled into three meals a day.

Never allow a baby to use a bottle of juice as a comforter or go to sleep with a bottle in his mouth, as this can result in serious tooth decay.

Sterilizing and Food Preparation

For babies older than six months, it isn't necesssary for the first solids to be completely smooth and soft, and you can start introducing some texture quite quickly, depending on your baby's preferences. Fork-mashing is simple and easy, but there are several useful pieces of kitchen equipment to help you with larger quantities.

For ease and speed, an electric liquidizer is by far the best. You may be able to buy a liquidizer attachment for your mixer, or purchase a free-standing liquidizer unit. A food processor works well, but make sure the food is blended to the required smoothness before offering it to your baby, as processors can miss the odd lump, especially when processing small quantities. A hand-held electric multimixer has the bonus of reducing washing up by mixing foods in the serving bowl. If you prefer to purée food by hand, then a sieve (strainer) or hand mill are both perfectly adequate and are much cheaper alternatives.

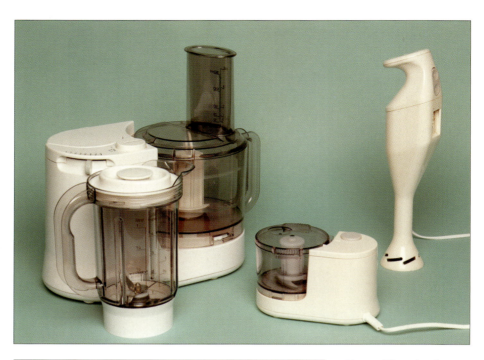

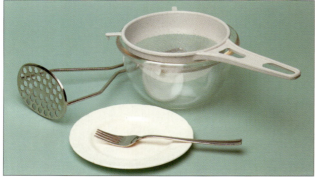

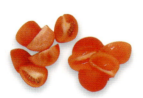

Above: *There is a huge range of brand-name food processors and blenders on the market, many of which have attachments for puréeing.*

Left: *The basics – manual mashers, or a sieve – take longer but will do the job just as well.*

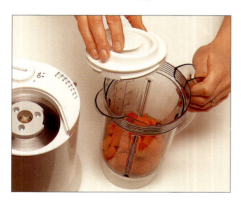

Above: *A purpose-designed liquidizer will make perfect purée in seconds. This is the right tool for making large batches.*

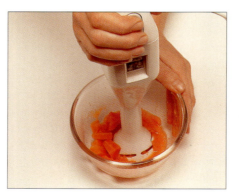

Above: *This hand-held blender takes a little longer, but the results are just as reliable. They are easy to clean and store.*

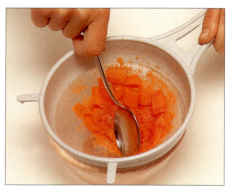

Above: *Making purée manually the old-fashioned way – with a sieve and spoon – is time-consuming but highly satisfying.*

FOOD HYGIENE

Young babies can easily pick up infections, so it is vitally important that all equipment is scrupulously clean before use.

● Always wash your hands before handling food or feeding equipment.

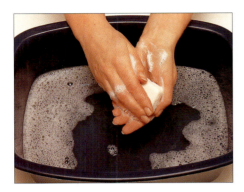

Above: *Rule one – always wash your hands with soap and warm water before feeding your baby or handling food.*

● Items such as bottles, feeding spoons and serving bowls should be sterilized until your baby is six-and-a-half months old. Sterilize equipment by boiling it in a pan of water for 25 minutes, immersing it in a container of cold water with sterilizing fluid or a tablet, or by using a steam sterilizer. Larger items such as a sieve, knife, pan, blender or masher, or plastic chopping board should be scalded with boiling water.

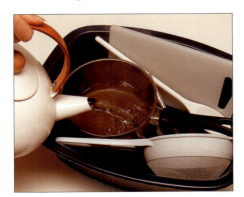

Above: *Scald larger objects such as chopping boards, spoons, sieves and pans with boiling water to sterilize.*

● Sterilize all baby equipment until your baby is six-and-a-half months; milk bottles, teats and so on should be sterilized until she begins to use a cup.

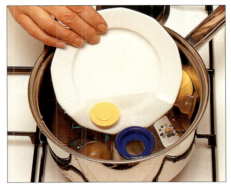

Above: *Boiling for 25 minutes is still the simplest way of sterilizing baby equipment.*

Right *Always cover baby food at all times – even when stored in the refrigerator.*

Below: *Always keep the surfaces around where your baby eats scrupulously clean.*

● Never use equipment used for the family pet when preparing baby food. Keep a can opener, fork and dish specifically for your pet, and make sure other members of the family are aware of this.

● Once cooked, cover all baby food with a lid or plate and transfer to the refrigerator as soon as possible. Food should not be left for longer than 1½ hours at room temperature before either refrigerating or freezing.

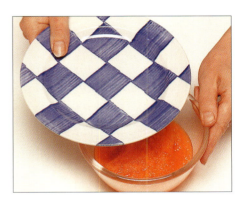

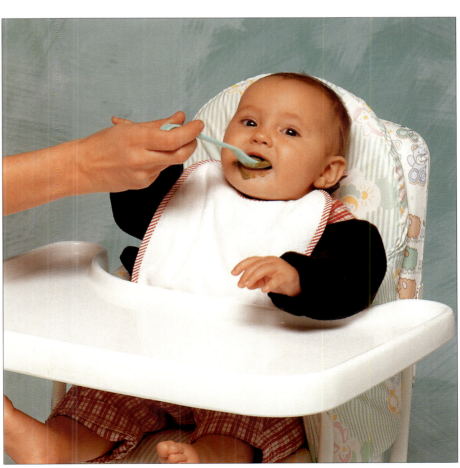

SOLUTION STERILIZER

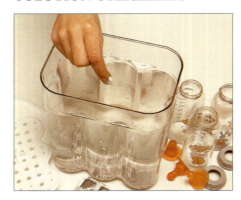

1 Fill the sterilizer to the required height with cold water, and add sterilizing tablets or liquid.

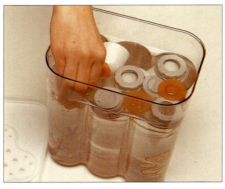

2 Pack the items to be sterilized into the container. Bottles will fit into the spaces provided.

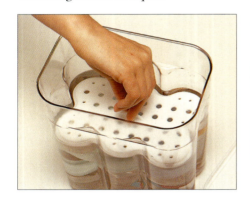

3 Make sure no air gets trapped in the container – or these pockets will not be properly sterile. Push everything down with the "float".

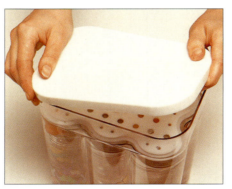

4 Place the lid on and leave for the length of time specified in the instructions. Rinse everything afterwards in boiling water.

STEAM STERILIZER

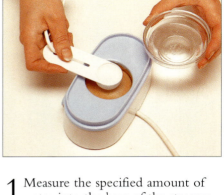

1 Measure the specified amount of water into the base of the steamer as directed in the instructions.

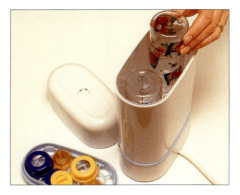

2 Pack the bottles and teats into the container: steamers have less capacity for dishes, which will need to be boiled separately.

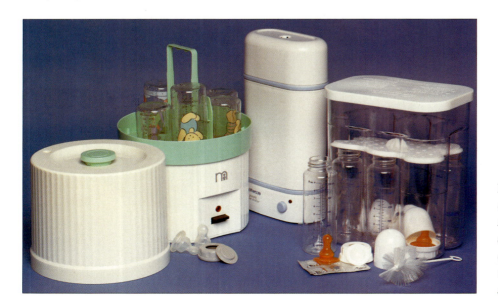

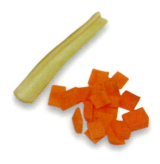

Left: *There is a wide range of sterilizing equipment to choose from. This group, all specially designed for bottles and teats, comprises two steam sterilizing units that operate electrically and a traditional container that holds the bottles efficiently in cold water sterilizing solution.*

STERILIZING IN THE MICROWAVE

Microwave ovens are not suitable for general day-to-day sterilizing without special equipment, and many health authorities and mother-and-baby experts recommend against using the microwave for this purpose. However, microwave sterilizing units can be purchased for sterilizing bottles, and if you are using one, the manufacturer's instructions should be followed closely.

Right: This purpose-designed sterilizing unit is specially made for microwave use. Add about 5mm/¹/₄in water to the base before putting in the bottles.

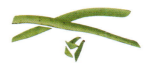

BATCH COOKING

Cooking for a baby can be very frustrating. Those spoonfuls of lovingly and hygienically prepared food, offered with such hope and spat out so unceremoniously can leave you feeling quite indignant.

Save time by cooking several meals in advance. Freeze mini-portions in ice-cube trays, great for those early days when you need only one cube for lunch, and flexible enough for later on when your baby's appetite has grown to two or three cubes per meal.

Spoon the mixture into sterilized ice-cube trays and open freeze until solid. Press the cubes into a plastic bag, seal, label and return to the freezer. Keep single batches of food in the same bag so that the different flavours don't combine.

Recycle yogurt containers, cottage cheese containers with lids, small plastic boxes with lids, or use disposable plastic cups and cover them with clear film (plastic wrap). Sterilize the containers using sterilizing fluid or tablets. Cover all prepared foods and label them clearly so that you know what they are and on which date they went into the freezer.

Most foods should be used within three months if stored in a freezer at – 18°C/0°F. Defrost plastic boxes in the refrigerator overnight. Ice cubes can be left to defrost at room temperature in a bowl or on a plate, loosely covered with clear film.

BATCH COOKING TIPS

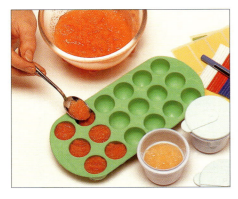

1 It is just as quick (and very much cheaper in the long run) to make a larger batch of purée as a smaller quantity for a single meal.

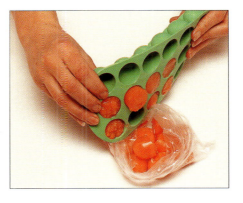

2 Freeze in meal-size portions in sterilized ice-cube trays: these can later be put into freezer bags for storing.

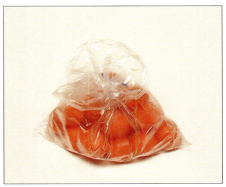

3 Make sure the bags are carefully labelled and dated. Keep only for the period specified in your freezer handbook.

Reheating, Freezing and Using a Microwave

HOW TO REHEAT BABY FOOD

Although reheating food sounds relatively straightforward, it is vitally important that the following rules are followed, as tepid food provides the perfect breeding ground for bacteria, especially if left uncovered in a warm kitchen and reheated several times.

● Don't reheat food more than once. It is a health risk, and can be dangerous.

● If you have a large batch of baby food, then reheat just a portion in a pan and leave the remaining mixture in a covered bowl in the refrigerator. If your baby is still hungry after the feed, then reheat a little extra again, with the remaining mixture left in the refrigerator.

● Reheat small quantities of baby food in a sterilized heat-proof container, covered with a saucer or small plate and put into a small pan half filled with boiling water. Alternatively, spoon larger quantities straight into a pan, cover and bring to the boil.

● Make sure food is piping hot all the way through to kill any bacteria. Food should be 70°C/158°F for a minimum of 2 minutes. Take off the heat and allow to cool. Test before serving to your baby.

REHEATING TIPS

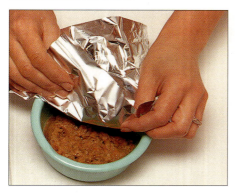

1 Reheat small quantities in a sterilized bowl, covered with a dish or foil.

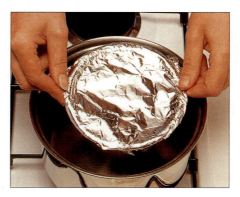

2 Place the bowl into a pan half filled with boiling water. Make sure the food is cooked through.

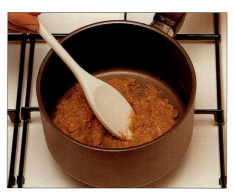

3 For larger quantities, put the food straight into the pan and bring to the boil.

FREEZING

● When using a freezer for storing home-made baby foods, use up the foods as soon as possible, as the texture preferred by the child will change very quickly as she develops.

● Keeping a well-stocked freezer of basic provisions can frequently be a real life-saver: there are few things worse than going shopping with small children, especially when they're tired, and freezing their food will save you trip after trip.

● Make sure that you always label foods that are going in the freezer. Labels will let you know exactly when they went into the freezer. Double check the dates against this handy list of storage dates:

Meat and poultry

Beef and lamb	4–6 months
Pork and veal	4–6 months
Minced (ground) beef	3–4 months
Sausages	2–3 months
Ham and bacon joints	3–4 months
Chicken and turkey	10–12 months
Duck and goose	4–6 months

Fish

White fish	6–8 months
Oily fish	3–4 months
Fish portions	3–4 months
Shellfish	2–3 months

Fruit and vegetables

Fruit with/without sugar	8–10 months
Fruit juices	4–6 months
Most vegetables	10–12 months
Mushrooms and tomatoes	6–8 months

Dairy produce

Cream	6–8 months
Butter, unsalted (sweet)	6–8 months
Butter, salted	3–4 months
Cheese, hard	4–6 months
Cheese, soft	3–4 months
Ice cream	3–4 months

Prepared foods

Ready-prepared meals, highly seasoned	2–3 months
Ready-prepared meals, average seasoning	4–6 months
Cakes	4–6 months
Bread, all kinds	2–3 months
Other yeast products and pastries	3–4 months

Chart published by kind permission of the Food Safety Advisory Centre

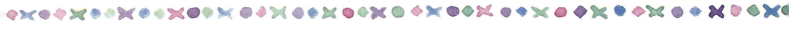

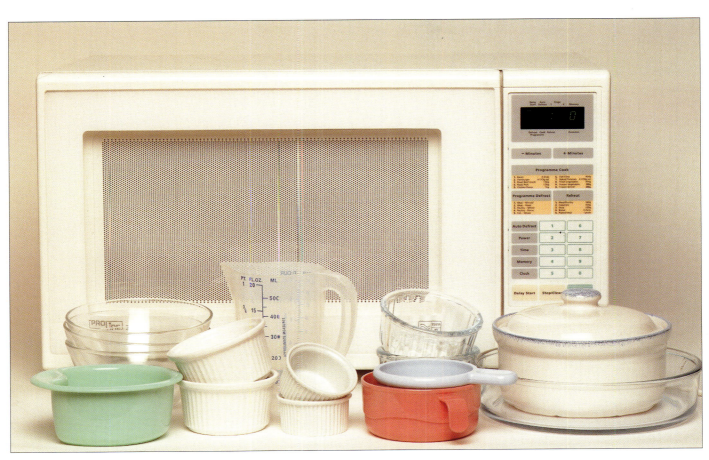

Above: *Many parents will find a microwave helpful and time-saving if used carefully. It can be used for heating milk and drinks (for toddlers – not newborns), for defrosting, reheating and cooking preprepared foods.*

USING A MICROWAVE

Health advisers do not recommend using a microwave for reheating, as the food heats up unevenly, but if you decide to microwave baby food, then make sure you stir the food thoroughly after cooking. Leave the dish to stand for 2–3 minutes before stirring again so that "hot spots" are well stirred into the mixture, and always check the temperature before serving. Choose the type of dish you use carefully as some ceramic dishes can get extremely hot; plastic or pyrex dishes are generally the most successful in the microwave, heating food quickly but staying relatively cool themselves.

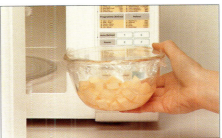

1 Cover with clear film (plastic wrap), pierce and place in the oven.

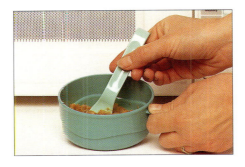

2 When cooked, remove from the microwave oven and stir.

MICROWAVING TIPS

● Never warm milk for a newborn or young baby in the microwave.

● For older children, warm milk in a bottle without the teat or in an uncovered feeder beaker for 30–45 seconds. Stir well and always test the temperature of the milk (*not* the temperature of the container) before serving to make sure that the milk is an even and comfortable temperature. Seek advice from your doctor or health visitor.

● To defrost ice cubes of baby food, press three into a baby dish, cover with clear film (plastic wrap) and thaw in the microwave on Defrost (30%) for 1–2 minutes. Stir well then re-cover and microwave on Full Power (100%) for 1 minute. Stir well to avoid hot spots, then test the temperature.

Choosing a High-chair

There is a surprisingly wide choice of high-chairs available in a range of finishes, colours and price levels, so make sure you shop around before you decide which style of chair to buy. Those shown here are just a selection of the many different chairs that are available.

CONVERTIBLE CHAIRS

Designed for babies between four weeks and six months, these chairs can convert from a high-chair into a swing, and some models will also convert into a baby chair and rocker too. It is best to buy one of these when the baby is very young so that you get maximum use from it. The only disadvantage may be the space required for the frame. The ease in converting from one type of chair to another varies from model to model, so you would be well advised to practise converting the chair in the shop before choosing which one to buy. Most chairs have white painted frames.

THREE-IN-ONE CHAIRS

Various designs on the market convert into a separate chair, chair and table or high-chair. Some simply clip apart, while others require a little help with a screwdriver. There are good rigid structures available with a wide range of decorative seat patterns. They are available in wood or white finishes. The low chair is suitable for children up to four years old if used without the tray.

ELEVATOR CHAIRS

These chairs are slightly more expensive, but will convert from a high-chair to a low chair. Some models have adjustable tray settings so that the tray can be moved to suit a growing child. The frames are mostly available in white metal, with attractive seating.

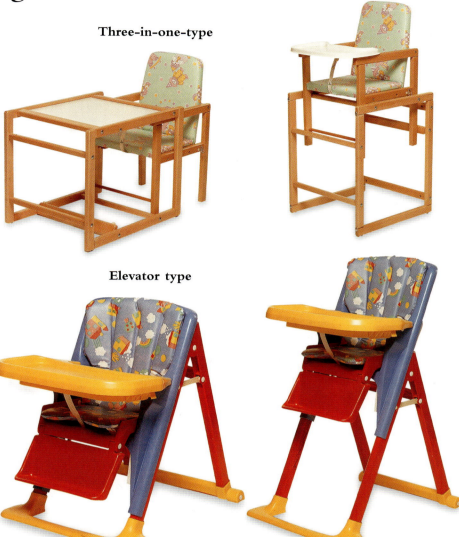

Three-in-one-type

Elevator type

TIPS

● For maximum use of a high-chair, buy a booster cushion for the early days when your baby first begins to use the chair. Adjust the tray position as well, if possible.
● Check that the high-chair is easy to clean – dried-on food in cracks can be impossible to clean off. Look out for possible dirt traps on the seat or around the tray fixing.
● Make sure that the chair is sturdy and rigid – it will need to withstand considerable wear.

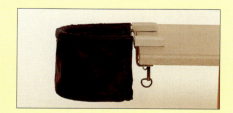

Above: *A portable clip-on chair.*

● If using a clip-on high-chair make sure that the table is suitable and will be able to withstand the weight of your child. Never, in any circumstances, fix on to glass.

FOLDING CHAIRS

These less expensive chairs, available in wood or white finishes, usually fold up in a scissor movement. Some can be folded crossways for packing into the boot (trunk) of the car. Before buying, check how easy they are to fold out and up, and make sure the frame is rigid when opened out.

Folding type

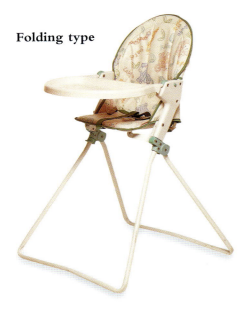

COUNTRY-TYPE CHAIRS

These are sturdy wooden high-chairs usually with a wooden tray and attractive spindle features. The seat can be hard for the baby, so it is best to buy a fitted chair cushion.

PORTABLE CHAIRS

There are two main types available:
● A very simple cloth tie, useful for visiting friends or eating out, as it will fold up and fit in a bag. However, it is not really suitable for everyday use as the child is literally tied on to the chair and so cannot reach the table to feed himself.
● Clip-on seats where the frames are placed under and over the edge of a dining table. Check that the table is strong enough and is not likely to overbalance before you put your baby in the chair.

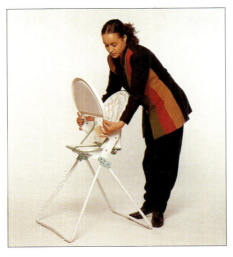

1 Undo the tray catches by pressing both sides at once, and fold the tray upwards.

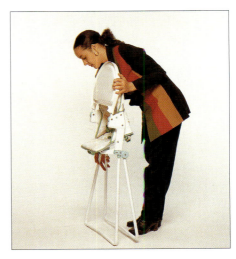

2 Undo the side catches that keep the frame rigid so the chair can scissor in two.

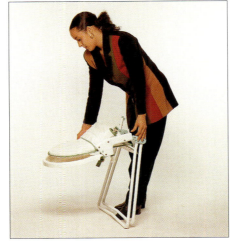

3 This allows you to fold the chair over on to itself: the design is incredibly neat and compact.

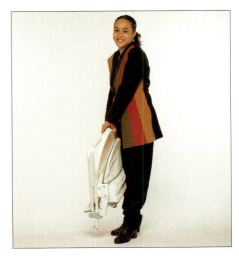

4 It is now ready for storing, putting out of the way, or placing in the boot (trunk) of the car.

TIPS
● Always use a safety harness. Although most high-chairs have a three-point lap strap, you will probably have to buy straps that will go around your baby's body and clip on to the chair. It is amazing how quickly a baby learns to wriggle out of a high-chair when you're not looking.
● Never leave a child in a high-chair unattended.

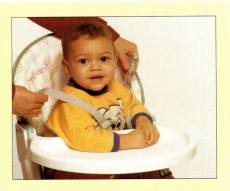

Above: *Always strap your baby in tightly.*

STAGE 1: FIRST TASTES – EARLY WEANING

OFFICIAL GUIDELINES NOW RECOMMEND THAT WEANING TAKES PLACE WHEN A BABY IS SIX OR SIX-AND-A-HALF MONTHS, BUT THERE ARE SOME BABIES WHO SHOW INTEREST IN EATING SOLIDS AT AN EARLIER AGE. YOU SHOULD NOT INTRODUCE SOLID FOODS BEFORE YOUR BABY IS 17 WEEKS OLD – AND BE SURE TO ASK YOUR DOCTOR OR HEALTH VISITOR FOR ADVICE BEFORE STARTING EARLY WEANING. BEGIN BY OFFERING ONLY A TEASPOONFUL OF BABY RICE OR SOME VERY SOFT RUNNY PURÉE ONCE A DAY. MILK IS STILL PROVIDING YOUR BABY WITH ALL HER NUTRITIONAL NEEDS, BUT THESE EARLY FOODS WILL BE THE FOUNDATIONS ON WHICH LATER EATING HABITS ARE BUILT, SO IT SHOULD BE A POSITIVE EXPERIENCE.

Suitable Foods

FOODS TO INCLUDE
- baby rice mixed with water, breast or formula milk
- mild-tasting fork-mashed vegetables – beginning with potato then carrot, parsnip, or swede (rutabaga)
- mild, naturally-sweet fruit purées made with eating apples or pears

Below: *If your baby seems ready to start taking solids at around four to five months old, start with a teaspoon and build gradually to two and finally three meals a day.*

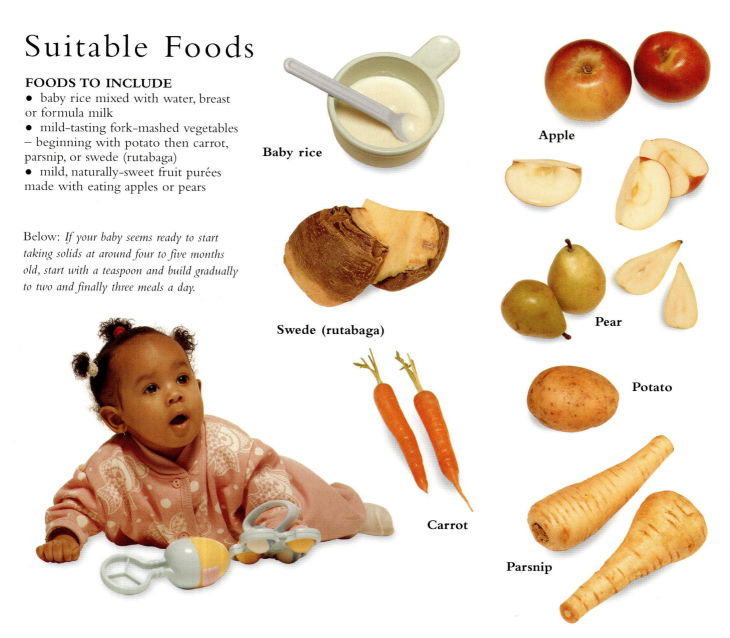

Baby rice

Apple

Swede (rutabaga)

Pear

Potato

Carrot

Parsnip

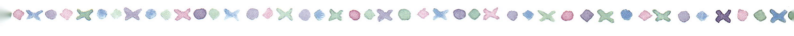

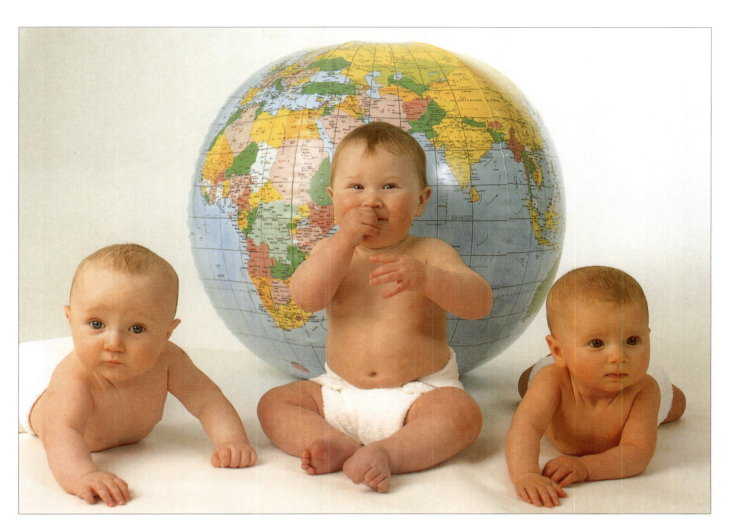

FOODS TO AVOID

- highly spiced foods
- salt as this causes the kidneys to overwork. Avoid seasoning with salt or adding stock cubes, bacon and salami to foods
- cows' milk (give breast or formula milk feeds instead)
- foods containing gluten, found in wheat, oats, rye and barley (check pack labels)
- eggs
- meat, fish, poultry
- citrus and berry fruits – can result in allergic reactions in some babies
- nuts, either whole or ground
- honey
- fatty foods

Note: If you have a family history of allergies, your doctor or health visitor may also advise you to avoid other foods. Check with them.

Above: *A world of foodstuffs opens up over the months: but introduce them gradually, and at the right time.*

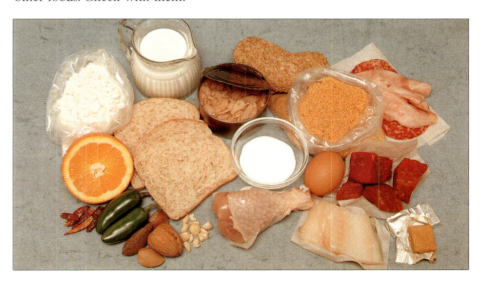

Right: *Adult favourites – but these must be avoided at this age, even as treats.*

Baby Rice

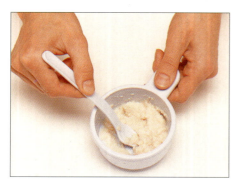

Mix 5-15ml/1-3 tsp rice with cooled boiled water, formula or breast milk as the pack directs. Cool slightly and test before serving.

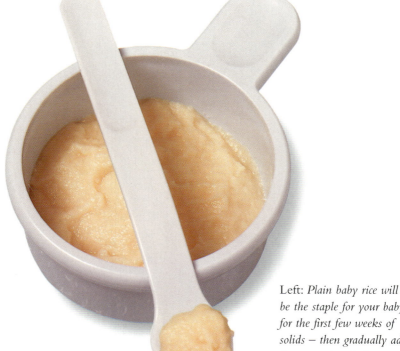

Left: *Plain baby rice will be the staple for your baby for the first few weeks of solids – then gradually add flavour and variation.*

Vegetable Purées

Makes: 175ml/6fl oz/¾ cup

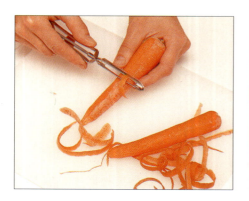

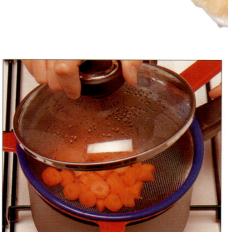

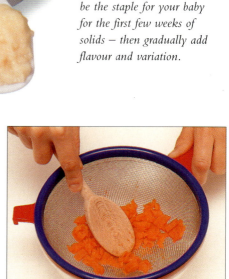

1 Peel 125g/3½oz potato, parsnip, carrot or swede (rutabaga) and chop into small dice.

• **To microwave**: put the vegetable or vegetables in a microwave-proof bowl with 30ml/2 tbsp formula or breast milk. Cover with clear film (plastic wrap), pierce and cook on Full Power (100%) for 4 minutes. Leave to stand for 5 minutes, then press through a sieve (strainer) and mix with 30–45ml/2–3 tbsp formula or breast milk. Cool and serve as above.

2 Steam over a pan of boiling water for 10 minutes, until soft.

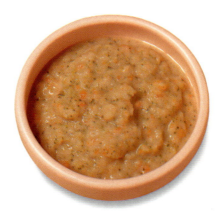

3 Press through a sieve (strainer), mix with 60–75ml/4–5 tbsp formula or breast milk, depending on the vegetable used. Spoon a little into a bowl, test on a spoon and cool if needed. Cover the remaining purée and transfer to the refrigerator as soon as possible. Use within 24 hours.

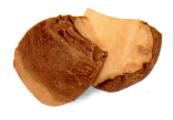

Fruit Purées

Makes: 120ml/4fl oz/½ cup

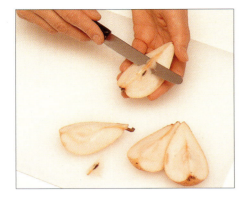

1 Peel, quarter and core 1 dessert apple or 1 ripe pear.

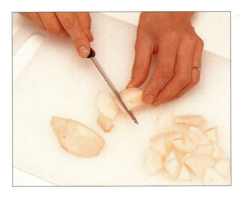

2 Thinly slice and put in a small pan with 15ml/1 tbsp water, formula or breast milk. Cover and simmer for 10 minutes, until soft.

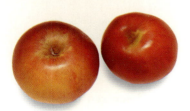

● **To microwave:** place the apple or pear in a microwave-proof bowl with water, formula or breast milk. Cover with clear film (plastic wrap), pierce and cook on Full Power (100%) for 3 minutes. Leave to stand for 5 minutes, then press through a sieve (strainer). Cool and serve as above.

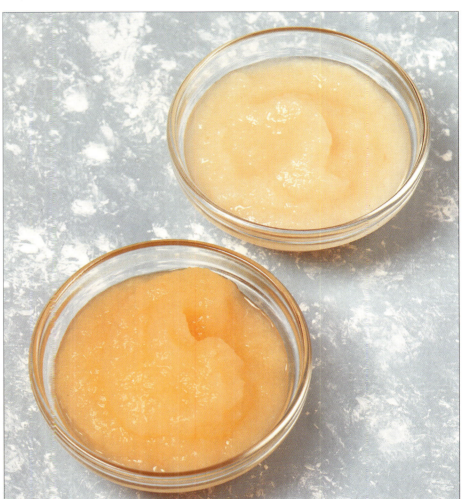

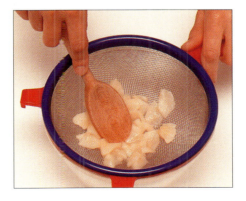

3 Press through a sieve (strainer). Spoon a little purée into a serving bowl, test on a spoon and cool if needed. Cover, transfer to the refrigerator, and use within 24 hours.

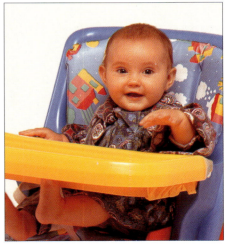

Top: *Pear and apple purée (top) will bring a smile to any baby's face (above).*

STAGE 2: AROUND SIX TO SIX-AND-A-HALF MONTHS

IF YOU BEGIN WEANING AT SIX MONTHS, START WITH BABY RICE AND RUNNY VEGETABLE AND FRUIT PURÉE. IF YOU HAVE ALREADY INTRODUCED YOUR BABY TO SOLIDS, INCREASE THE VARIETY OF FOODS OFFERED AND START TO COMBINE FOOD TASTES. PURÉE CAN BE A THICKER COARSER TEXTURE, BUT MAKE SURE THERE ARE NO PIPS (SEEDS) OR BONES. ALWAYS CHOOSE THE BEST, FRESHEST INGREDIENTS AND MAKE SURE UTENSILS ARE SCRUPULOUSLY CLEAN.

Suitable Foods

FOODS TO INCLUDE

● wide selection of vegetables, including fresh or frozen peas, corn, cauliflower, broccoli, cabbage, spinach, celery, mushrooms and leeks
● fruits – banana, apricots, peaches, plums, strawberries, raspberries, melon (Warning: offer tiny amounts of soft berry fruits as some children may be allergic to them.)
● chicken
● mild-tasting fresh or frozen fish – plaice, cod, haddock, trout
● small quantities of very lean red meat
● small quantities of split peas and red lentils, and very well-cooked or canned whole chickpeas and beans
● gluten-free cereals – rice, cornflour (cornstarch)

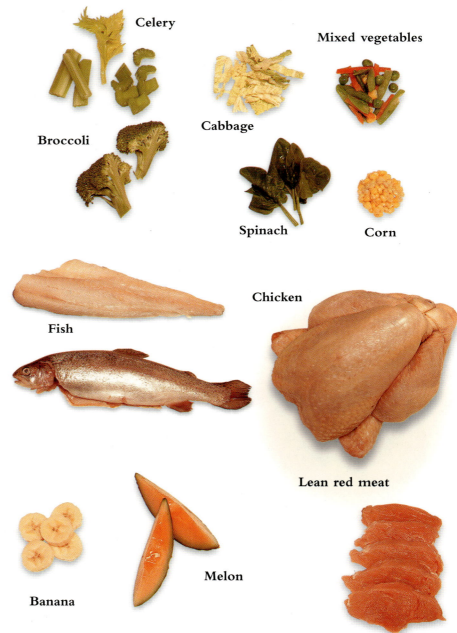

Celery

Mixed vegetables

Cabbage

Broccoli

Spinach

Corn

Fish

Chicken

Lean red meat

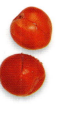

Plums

Apricots

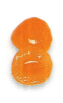

Banana

Melon

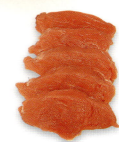

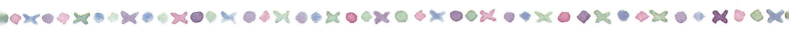

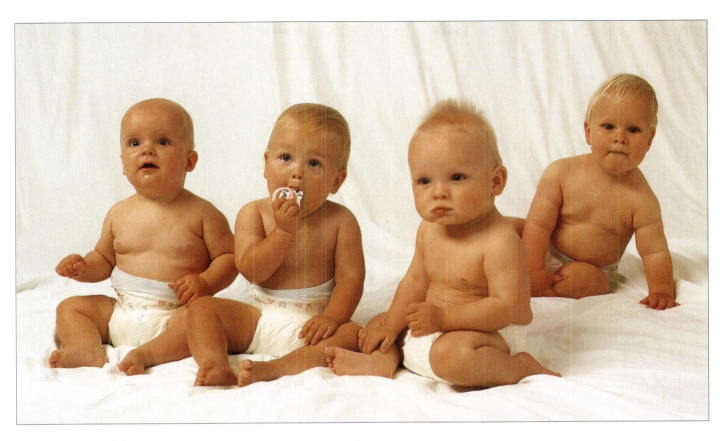

Above: *Every day brings a new taste: these young gourmets can't wait!*

FOODS TO AVOID

- gluten–based cereals, wheat flour and bread
- cow's milk and milk products
- eggs
- citrus and berry fruits
- nuts, ground or whole
- honey
- fatty foods
- salt and highly spiced foods

Below: *Even healthy adult foods such as wholewheat bread and oranges should be avoided.*

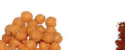

Chickpeas   **Cocoa**

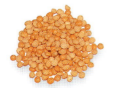

Split peas   **Cornflour (cornstarch)**

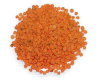

Lentils   **Rice**

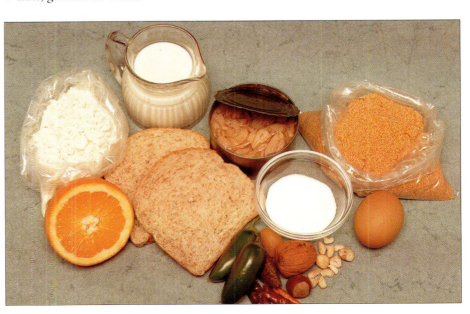

Going Vegetarian

A vegetarian diet can provide all the necessary nutrients for health and vitality, but it is important to balance the baby's diet to ensure that she receives adequate supplies of protein, vitamins D and B12, calcium and iron.

The basic guidelines are the same as for weaning any other baby: introduce flavours slowly and be guided by your baby. The biggest differences are obviously in the type of foods offered. Instead of obtaining protein from meat and fish, your baby will receive it from other protein-rich food. These include eggs, beans, peas, split lentils, and grains, finely ground nuts or nut creams, sunflower seed spread, milk and dairy products, and vegetarian cheese where available.

Vegetarians need to make sure that sufficient iron is included in their baby's diet. If she is over six months, offer prune juice, puréed apricots, molasses, refined lentils and cereals, particularly fortified breakfast cereals. Green vegetables and well-mashed beans, if over eight months, are also a good source of iron. Vitamin C aids the absorption of iron from plant sources, so make sure you serve fresh green vegetables or fruit in the meal. Your doctor may also think it is beneficial for your baby to take vitamin drops.

If you plan to bring the baby up as a vegan and so omit dairy products and eggs from the diet, then it is vital to consult your doctor or dietician.

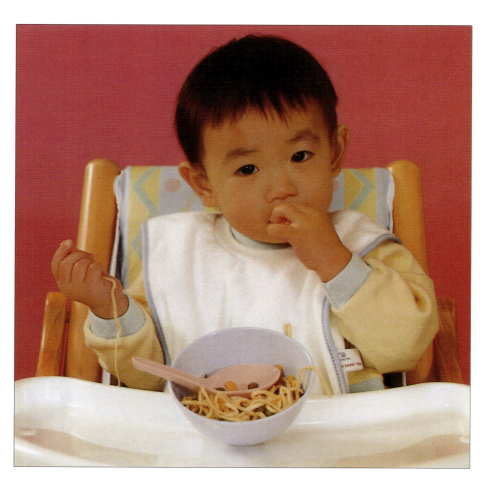

Vegetarian diets tend to be bulky and lower in calories than a diet containing meat, so make sure you include foods that are protein and calorie rich, with little or no fibre, such as eggs, milk and cheese. These can be mixed with smaller quantities of vegetables, fruit and cereals. Fibre-rich foods can also be difficult for a child to digest as many nutrients

Above: *Raising your child as a vegetarian takes special planning and care to make sure all the necessary nutrients are included.*

may pass straight through the body. To ensure your baby is getting the correct amount of vitamins, minerals and food energy her diet should include foods from the four groups on the opposite page.

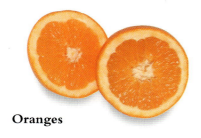

Oranges

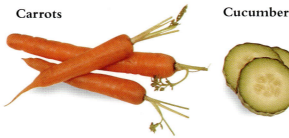

Carrots

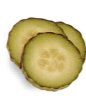

Cucumber

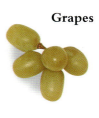

Grapes

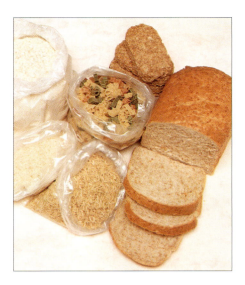

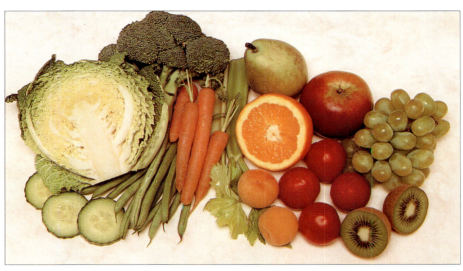

Cereals and grains: baby rice no earlier than 17 weeks; pasta, bread, oats and breakfast cereals from 6 months.

Fruit and vegetables: begin with potato, carrot, apple and pear at 6 to 6½ months, progressing to stronger-flavoured foods such as broccoli, beans, oranges and plums as your baby develops.

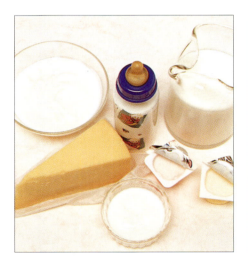

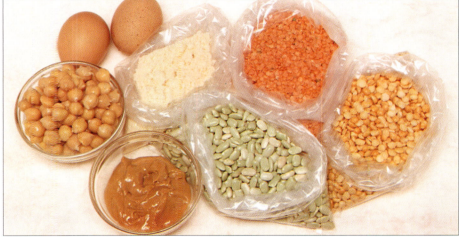

Dairy produce: including milk, cheese, fromage frais and yogurt from 6 months.
Note: Make sure cheese is rennet-free. If you are unsure, ask the delicatessen assistant, or check the packet if pre-packed.

Beans, peas and lentils: split and softly cooked lentils from 6–6½ months. Gradual introduction of tofu, smooth peanut butter, hard-boiled egg from 6 months. Well-cooked, mashed dried beans and peas and finely ground nuts from 9 months. Do not give whole nuts to the under-5s.

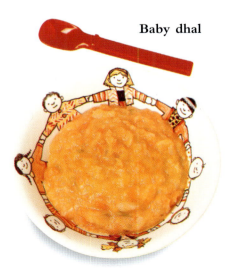

Baby dhal

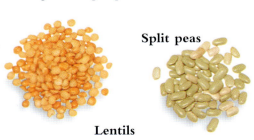

Split peas

Lentils

WEIGHT CHECK

To make sure your baby is thriving and happy, irrespective of the type of diet, you should visit a health clinic at regular intervals for a weight check.

Autumn Harvest

Makes: 600ml/1 pint/2½ cups

115g/4oz carrot

115g/4oz parsnip

115g/4oz swede (rutabaga)

115g/4oz potato

300ml/½ pint/1¼ cups formula milk

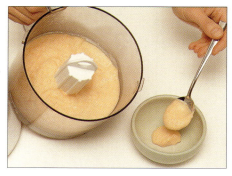

4 Spoon a little into a bowl. Test the temperature and cool if necessary, before giving to the baby.

5 Cover the remaining food and transfer to the refrigerator as soon as possible. Use within 24 hours.

• Suitable for freezing.

TIP
Thin the purée down with a little extra formula milk if your baby prefers a very soft purée.

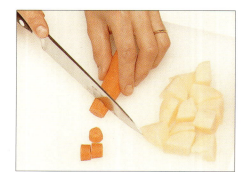

1 Trim and peel the carrot, parsnip, swede and potato, and place in a colander. Rinse under cold water, drain and chop.

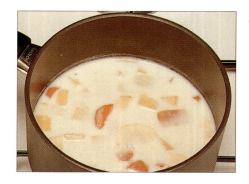

2 Place the chopped vegetables in a pan with the formula milk, then bring to the boil, cover and simmer for 20 minutes, or until they are very soft.

3 Purée, mash or sieve (strain) the vegetables until they are smooth.

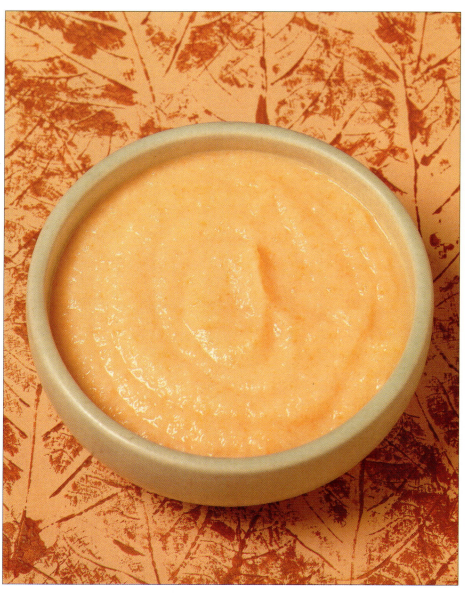

Mixed Vegetable Platter

Makes: 600ml/1 pint/2½ cups

115g/4oz carrot

175g/6oz potato

115g/4oz broccoli

50g/2oz green cabbage

300ml/½ pint/1¼ cups formula milk

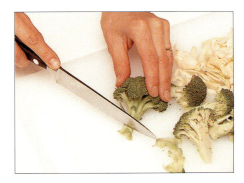

1 Peel the carrot and potato. Rinse, chop and place in a pan. Wash the broccoli and cabbage and cut the broccoli into florets and the stems into thin slices. Shred the cabbage finely.

2 Add the milk to the carrot and potato, bring to the boil, then cover and simmer for 10 minutes.

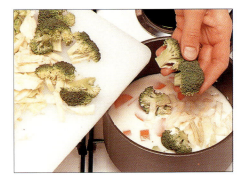

3 Add the broccoli stems and florets and cabbage, and cook, covered, for 10 minutes, until all the vegetables are tender.

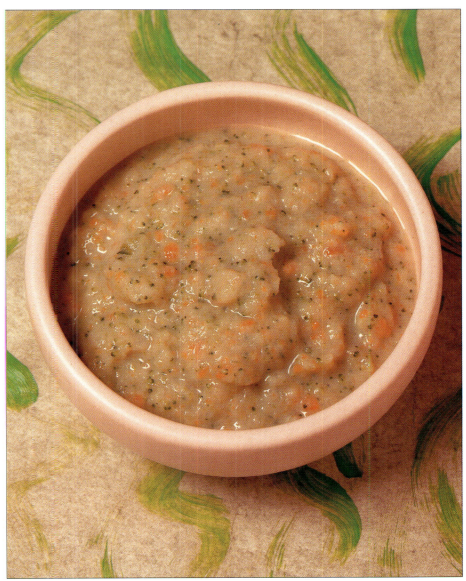

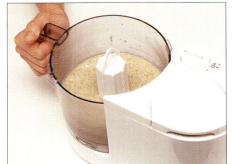

5 Spoon a little into a bowl. Test the temperature and cool if necessary, before giving to the baby.

6 Cover the remaining food and transfer to the refrigerator as soon as possible. Use within 24 hours.

• Suitable for freezing.

4 Purée, mash or sieve (strain) the vegetables until smooth.

Carrot, Lentil and Coriander Purée

Makes: 600ml/1 pint/2½ cups

350g/12oz carrots

175g/6oz potato

50g/2oz/¼ cup red lentils

2.5ml/½ tsp ground coriander

300ml/½ pint/1¼ cups formula milk

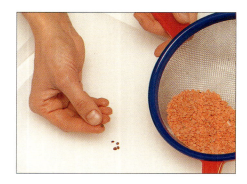

1 Trim and peel the carrots and potatoes and then chop into small cubes and place in a pan. Rinse the lentils thoroughly, discarding any black bits.

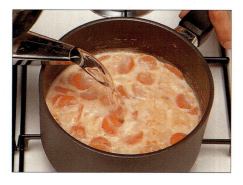

2 Add the lentils, coriander and milk to the pan and bring to the boil, then cover and simmer for 40 minutes, until the lentils are very soft. Top up with a little extra boiling water if necessary.

TIP

The mixture thickens on cooling so any remaining mixture will need to be thinned slightly with a little formula milk before reheating for the next meal.

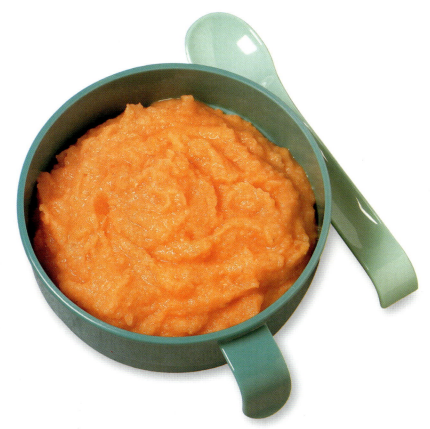

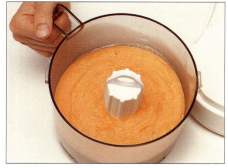

3 Purée, mash or sieve (strain) the mixture until smooth.

4 Spoon a little into a bowl. Test the temperature and cool if necessary, before giving to the baby.

5 Cover the remaining purée and transfer to the refrigerator as soon as possible. Use within 24 hours.

• Suitable for freezing.

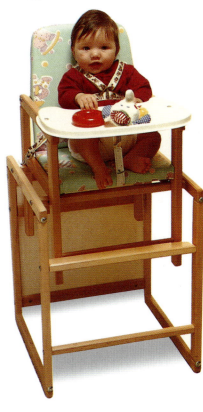

Red Pepper Risotto

Makes: 600ml/1 pint/2½ cups

50g/2oz/¼ cup long grain rice

300ml/½ pint/1¼ cups formula milk

75g/3oz red (bell) pepper

75g/3oz courgette (zucchini)

50g/2oz celery

1 Place the rice and milk in a pan, bring to the boil and simmer, uncovered, for 5 minutes.

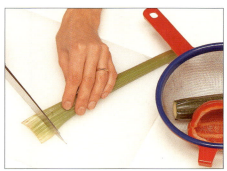

2 Discard the core and seeds from the pepper and trim the courgette and celery. Place the vegetables in a colander and rinse under cold water, then chop them into small pieces.

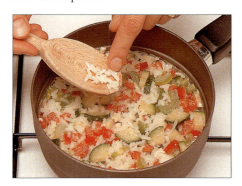

3 Add the vegetables to the rice mixture, bring to the boil, cover and simmer for about 10 minutes, or until the rice is soft.

• Suitable for freezing.

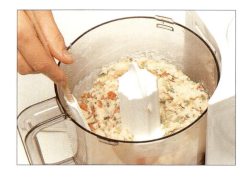

4 Purée, mash or sieve (strain) the rice mixture until smooth.

5 Spoon a little into a bowl. Test the temperature and cool if necessary before giving to the baby.

6 Cover the remaining food and transfer to the refrigerator as soon as possible. Use within 24 hours.

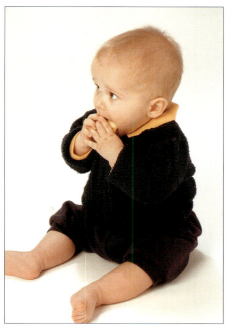

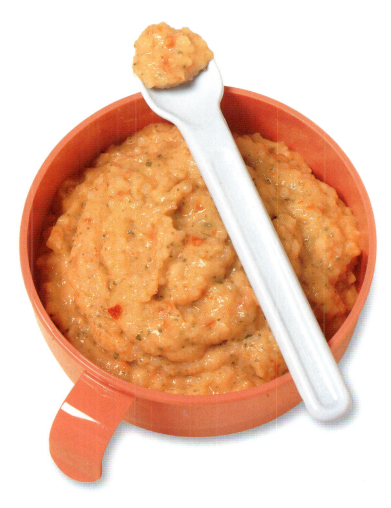

Parsnip and Broccoli Mix

Makes: 600ml/1 pint/2½ cups

225g/8oz parsnips

115g/4oz broccoli

300ml/½ pint/1¼ cups formula milk

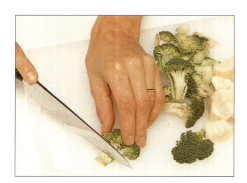

1 Trim and peel the parsnips and place in a colander with the broccoli. Rinse the parsnips and broccoli under cold water. Chop the parsnips and cut the broccoli into florets, slicing the stems.

2 Put the parsnips in a pan with the milk, bring to the boil, then cover and simmer for about 10 minutes.

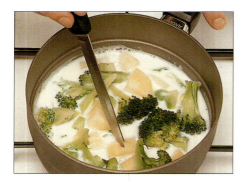

3 Add the broccoli and simmer for a further 10 minutes, until the vegetables are soft.

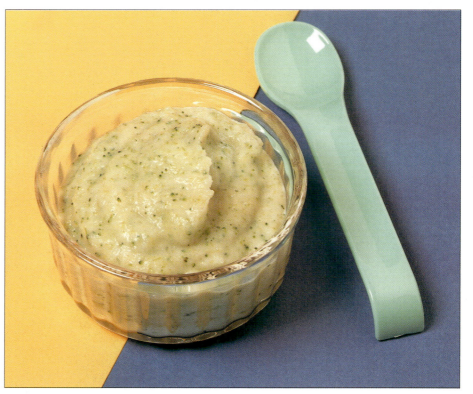

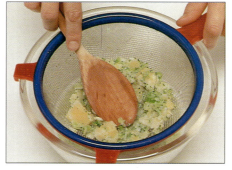

4 Purée, mash or sieve (strain) the vegetable mixture to make a completely smooth purée.

5 Spoon a little into a bowl. Test the temperature and cool if necessary, before giving to the baby.

6 Cover the remaining purée and transfer to the refrigerator as soon as possible. Use within 24 hours.

● Suitable for freezing.

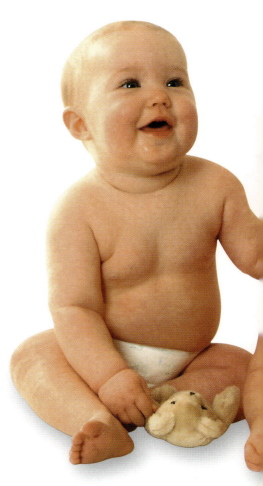

Turkey Stew with Carrots and Corn

Makes: 600ml/1 pint/2½ cups

175g/6oz potato

175g/6oz carrot

115g/4oz turkey breast, skinned and boned

50g/2oz/⅓ cup frozen corn

300ml/½ pint/1¼ cups formula milk

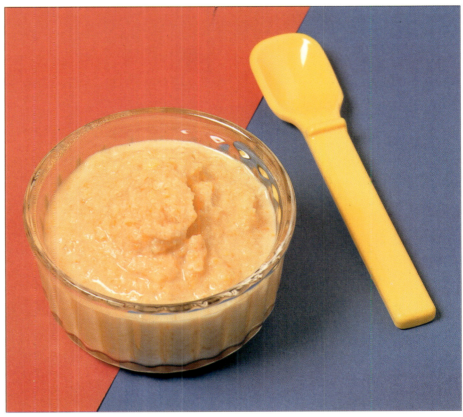

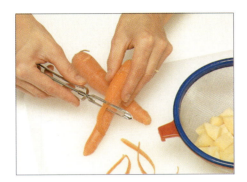

1 Trim and peel the potato and carrots, rinse under cold water and then chop into small cubes.

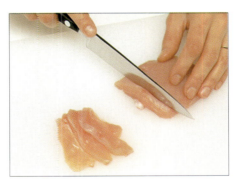

2 Rinse the turkey and cut into thin strips. Place in a small pan with the potato and carrot.

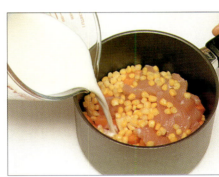

3 Add the corn and milk. Cover and simmer for 20 minutes, until the turkey is cooked. Purée, mash or sieve (strain) the mixture until smooth.

4 Spoon a little into a bowl. Test the temperature and cool if necessary, before giving to the baby.

5 Cover the remaining food and refrigerate. Use within 24 hours.

• Suitable for freezing.

TIP

Bring the mixture to the boil in a flameproof casserole and transfer to a preheated oven 180°C/350°F/ Gas 4 and cook for 1¼ hours if preferred.

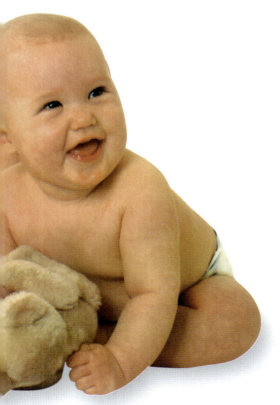

Chicken and Parsnip Purée

Makes: 600ml/1 pint/2½ cups

350g/12oz parsnips

115g/4oz chicken breast, skinned and boned

300ml/½ pint/1¼ cups formula milk

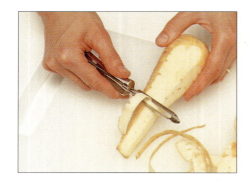

1 Peel the parsnips, and trim the woody tops and bottoms. Rinse and chop roughly.

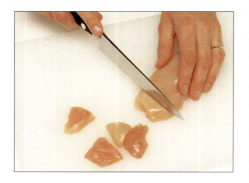

2 Rinse the chicken under cold water and cut into small pieces.

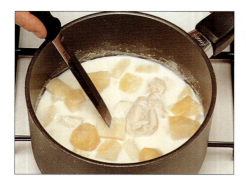

3 Place the parsnips, chicken and milk in a pan. Cover and simmer for 20 minutes, or until the parsnips are tender.

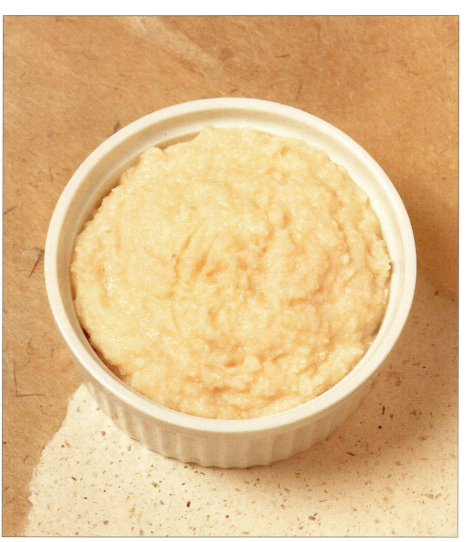

4 Purée, mash or sieve (strain) the mixture until smooth.

5 Spoon into a bowl. Test the temperature and cool if necessary, before giving to the baby.

6 Cover the remaining purée and transfer to the refrigerator as soon as possible. Use within 24 hours.

• Suitable for freezing.

TIP
For a very smooth purée, drain all the liquid into a liquidizer and add half the solids, blend until smooth, then add the remaining ingredients. If using a food processor, add all the solids and a little liquid, process until smooth, then add the remaining liquid.

Cock-a-Leekie Casserole

Makes: 600ml/1 pint/2½ cups

50g/2oz leek

275g/10oz potatoes

115g/4oz chicken breast, skinned and boned

300ml/½ pint/1¼ cups formula milk

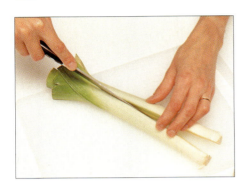

1 Halve the leek lengthways and rinse under running water to remove any dirt or grit.

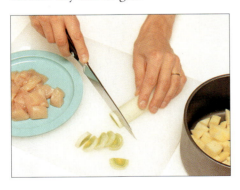

2 Peel potatoes and cut into small dice. Rinse the chicken and cut into pieces and thinly slice the leek.

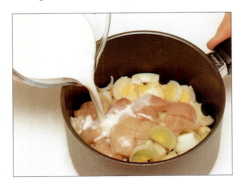

3 Place the vegetables and chicken in a pan with the milk.

4 Bring the mixture to the boil, cover with a lid and simmer gently for 20 minutes, until the potatoes are just tender. Purée, mash or sieve (strain) the mixture until it is completely smooth.

5 Spoon a little into a bowl. Test the temperature and cool if necessary, before giving to the baby. Use within 24 hours.

● Suitable for freezing.

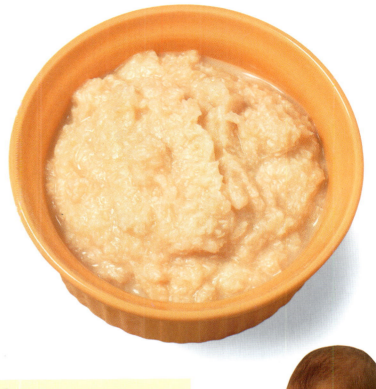

TIP
You can vary the texture of this recipe depending on how you purée the mixture. A fine sieve (strainer) produces the finest consistency, then a food processor, while a food mill gives the coarsest texture. Starchy vegetables thicken the purée and bind it together. Any root vegetable can be used for this recipe, but make sure it is thoroughly cooked before blending.

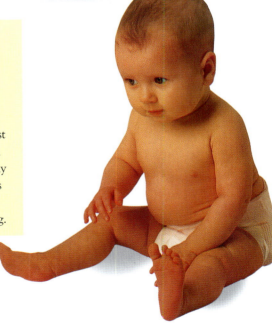

Trout and Courgette Savoury

Makes: 600ml/1 pint/2½ cups

275g/10oz potatoes

175g/6oz courgettes (zucchini)

115g/4oz pink trout fillet

250ml/8fl oz/1 cup formula milk

1 Peel the potatoes, trim the courgettes and rinse under cold water. Dice the potatoes and cut the courgettes into slices.

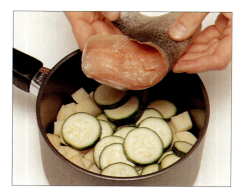

2 Place the vegetables in a pan. Rinse the trout and arrange on top, then pour over the milk. Bring to the boil, cover and simmer for 15 minutes, until the potatoes and fish are cooked.

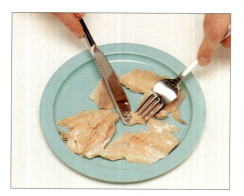

3 Lift the trout out of the pan and peel off the skin. Break it into pieces with a knife and fork, checking carefully for any bones.

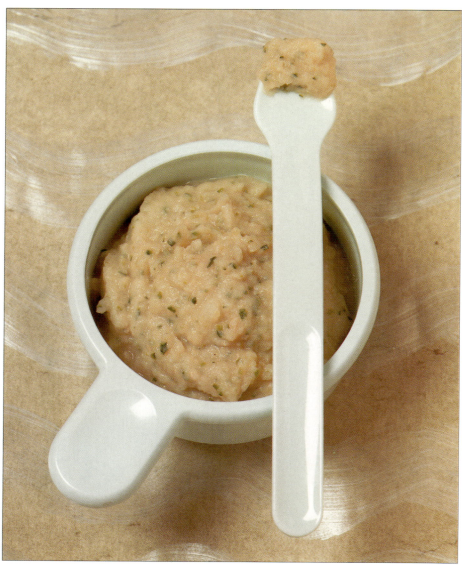

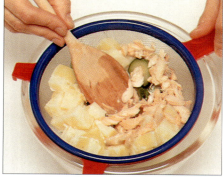

4 Purée, mash or sieve (strain) the fish, the vegetables and the liquid until quite smooth.

5 Spoon a little into a bowl. Test the temperature and cool if necessary, before giving to the baby.

6 Cover any remaining food and transfer to the refrigerator as soon as possible. Use within 24 hours.

• Suitable for freezing.

Fisherman's Pie

Makes: 600ml/1 pint/2½ cups

350g/12oz potatoes

90g/3½oz brick frozen skinless cod

25g/1oz/¼ cup frozen peas

25g/1oz/2 tbsp frozen corn

300ml/½ pint/1¼ cups formula milk

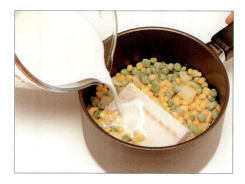

1 Peel and rinse the potatoes and cut into even pieces. Place in a pan with the fish, peas, corn and milk.

2 Bring to the boil, cover and simmer for 15 minutes, until the potatoes are very tender.

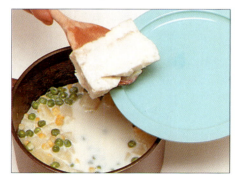

3 Lift the fish out of the pan and break into pieces with a knife and fork, checking carefully and removing any small bones.

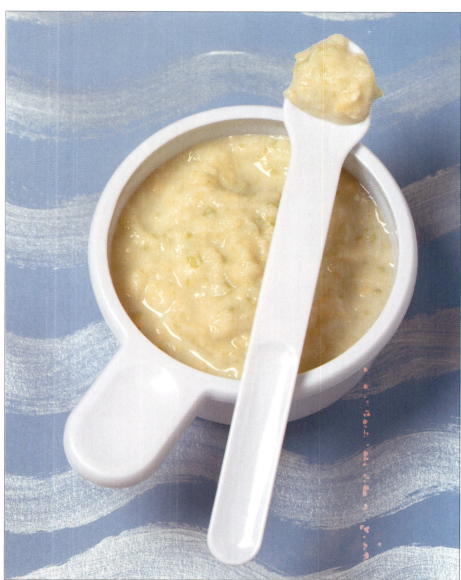

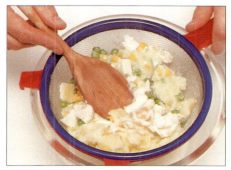

4 Purée, mash or sieve (strain) the fish, vegetables and cooking liquid until completely smooth.

5 Spoon a little into a bowl. Test the temperature and cool if necessary, before giving to the baby.

6 Cover the remaining purée and place in the refrigerator as soon as possible. Use within 24 hours.

• Suitable for freezing.

Apple Ambrosia

Makes: 300ml/½ pint/1¼ cups

1 eating apple

25g/1oz flaked rice

300ml/½ pint/1¼ cups formula milk

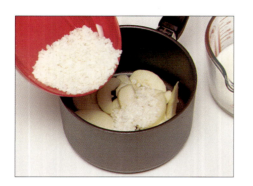

1 Quarter, core and peel the apple. Slice thinly and place in a pan with the rice and milk.

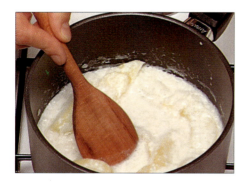

2 Bring to the boil then simmer over a gentle heat for 10–12 minutes, until the rice is soft, stirring occasionally with a wooden spoon.

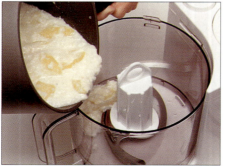

3 Purée or mash the apple and rice mixture until completely smooth.

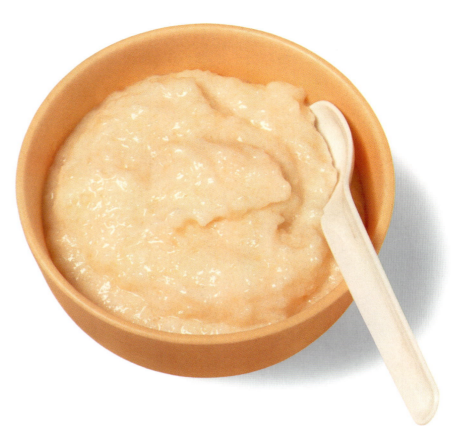

4 Spoon into a bowl. Test the temperature and cool if necessary, before giving to the baby. Cover the remaining purée and transfer to the refrigerator as soon as possible. Use within 24 hours.

VARIATION
Chocolate Pudding
Cook the rice as above but without the apple. Stir 25g/1oz milk chocolate dots and 15ml/1 tbsp caster (superfine) sugar into the hot rice and then purée or mash until smooth. Spoon into small dishes and cool as necessary.

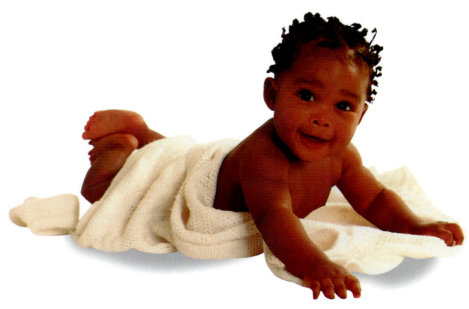

Fruit Salad Purée

Makes: 350ml/12fl oz/1½ cups

1 nectarine or peach

1 dessert apple

1 ripe pear

25g/1oz fresh or frozen raspberries
   or strawberries

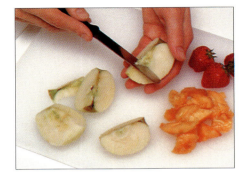

1 Halve the nectarine or peach, discard the stone (pit), then peel and chop. Peel, quarter and core the apple and pear and slice thinly.

2 Put the prepared fruits, the hulled raspberries or strawberries and 15ml/1 tbsp water in a pan. Cover and simmer for 10 minutes, until the fruit is soft.

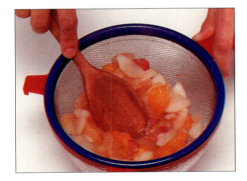

3 Press the mixture through a sieve (strainer) or process and then sieve (strain) to remove the berry pips (seeds). Discard the pips.

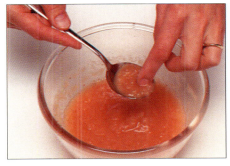

4 Spoon a little into a baby bowl. Test the temperature and cool if necessary, before giving to the baby.

5 Cover the remaining purée and transfer to the refrigerator as soon as possible. Use within 24 hours.

● Suitable for freezing.

TIP
Babies tend to eat smaller quantities of dessert, so it is best to open freeze purée in a sterilized ice cube tray. Transfer the cubes to a plastic bag once frozen.

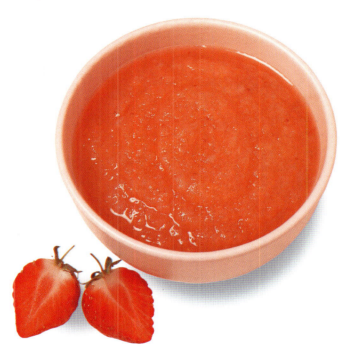

VARIATION
Peach and Melon Blush
To make 175ml/6fl oz/¾ cup, take 1 ripe peach and ¼ ripe Charentais melon. Peel and halve the peach, discard the stone (pit) and cut up the fruit. Scoop the seeds out of the melon and cut away the skin. Roughly chop the melon into pieces.
   Purée or sieve (strain) the fruit until completely smooth. Spoon a little into a bowl and serve.

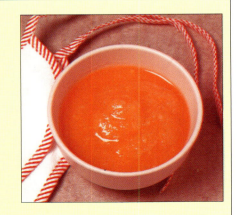

STAGE 3: SEVEN TO NINE MONTHS

FROM SEVEN TO NINE MONTHS IS A RAPID DEVELOPMENT PERIOD FOR YOUR BABY. BY EIGHT MONTHS, BABIES ARE USUALLY QUITE GOOD AT HOLDING THINGS, SO LET YOUR BABY HOLD A SECOND SPOON WHILE YOU ARE FEEDING HER, TO HELP DEVELOP CO-ORDINATION. THIS IS THE FIRST STEP TOWARDS SELF-FEEDING. ALL THE RECIPES FROM THE PREVIOUS SECTION CAN STILL BE MADE FOR YOUR GROWING BABY; JUST ADJUST THE TEXTURE SO THAT FOODS ARE SLIGHTLY COARSER.

Suitable Foods

FOODS TO INCLUDE
- wheat-based foods, pasta, bread – first fingers (thin slices) of toast or bread sticks
- breakfast cereals such as those made up with cows' milk
- cow's milk and dairy foods, e.g. yogurt, cottage cheese, mild Cheddar and Edam cheese
- red meat, but make sure you trim off fat and gristle
- hard-boiled egg yolk
- citrus fruits
- fingers of cooked carrot, broccoli
- smooth peanut butter

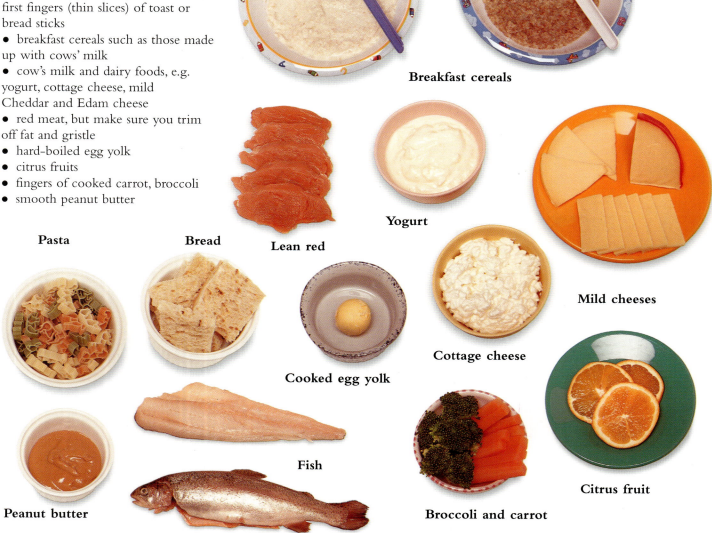

Breakfast cereals

Yogurt

Mild cheeses

Pasta   **Bread**

Lean red

Cottage cheese

Cooked egg yolk

Fish

Citrus fruit

Peanut butter

Broccoli and carrot

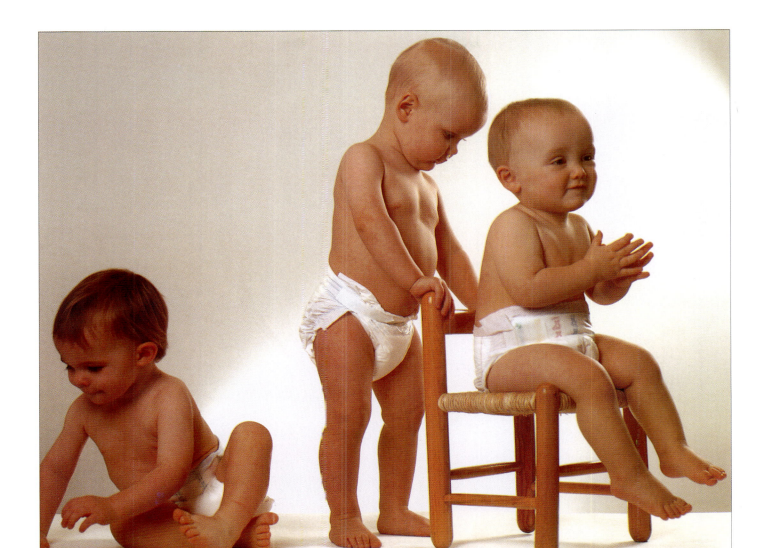

Above: *From seven to nine months your baby will develop rapidly.*

FOODS TO AVOID
- egg white
- whole or chopped nuts
- canned fish in brine
- organ meats – liver, kidney
- chillies and other very spicy foods
- salty foods
- sugary foods

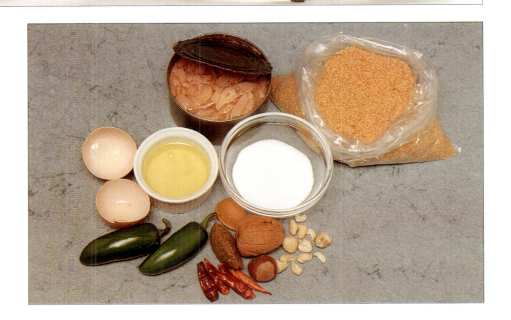

Right: *There is still a wide range of fatty, salty and spicy foods that must be avoided.*

Shepherd's Pie

Makes: 600ml/1 pint/2½ cups

2 tomatoes

¼ onion

225g/8oz potato

50g/2oz button (white) mushrooms

115g/4oz lean minced (ground) beef

250ml/8fl oz/1 cup water

15ml/1 tbsp tomato ketchup

pinch of dried mixed herbs

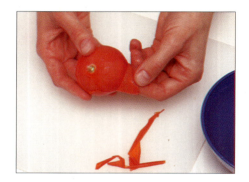

1 Make a cross cut in each tomato, put in a small bowl and cover with boiling water. Leave to stand for 1 minute and then drain and peel off the skins. Cut into quarters and scoop out the seeds.

2 Finely chop the onion, chop the potato and slice the mushrooms.

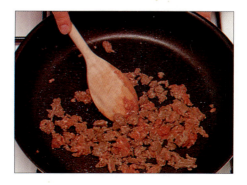

3 Dry-fry the beef in a pan for 5 minutes, stirring until browned all over.

• Suitable for freezing.

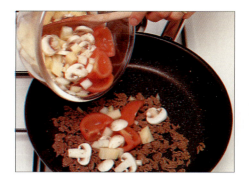

4 Add the tomatoes, potato, mushrooms and onion and cook for a further 3 minutes. Stir well to blend all the flavours together.

5 Add the water, ketchup and herbs. Bring to the boil, then reduce the heat, cover and simmer for 40 minutes, until the meat and vegetables are tender.

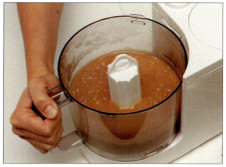

6 Process or mash the meat and vegetables just enough to give the desired consistency.

7 Spoon a little into a bowl. Test the temperature and cool if necessary, before giving to the baby.

8 Cover the remainder and refrigerate. Use within 24 hours.

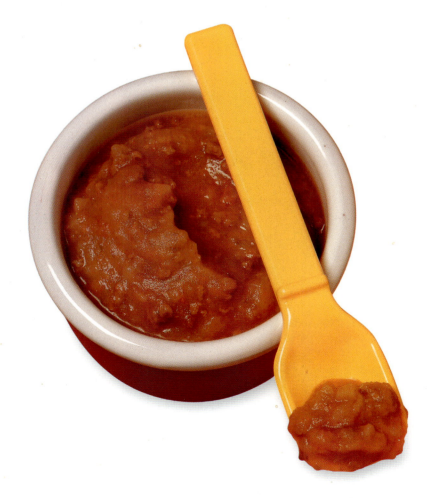

Braised Beef and Carrots

Makes: 600ml/1 pint/2½ cups

175g/6oz potato
225g/8oz carrots
¼ onion
175g/6oz stewing beef
300ml/½ pint/1¼ cups water
pinch of dried mixed herbs

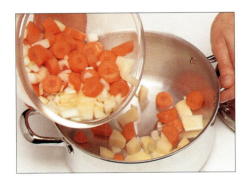

1 Preheat the oven to 180°C/350°F/Gas 4. Peel and chop the potato, carrots and onion, and place in a flameproof casserole.

2 Rinse the beef, cut away any fat and gristle and cut into small cubes using a sharp knife.

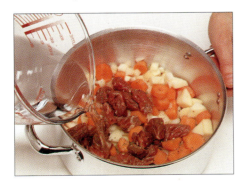

3 Add the meat, water and herbs to the casserole, bring to the boil and then cover and cook in the oven for 1½ hours, or until the meat is tender and the vegetables are soft.

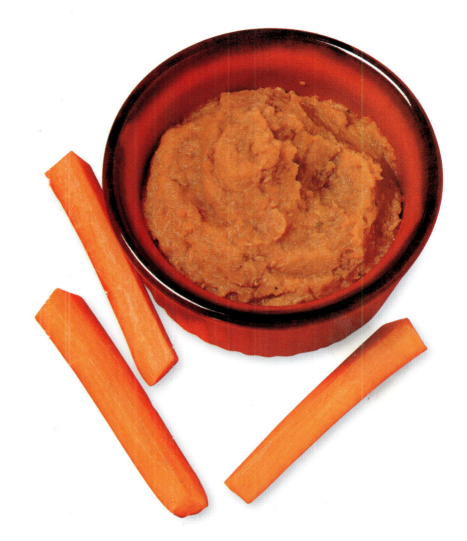

4 Process or mash the ingredients to the desired consistency and spoon a little into a bowl. Test the temperature and cool if necessary, before giving to the baby.

5 Cover any unused food and transfer to the refrigerator as soon as possible. Use within 24 hours.

• Suitable for freezing.

TIP
Replace the carrots with any other root vegetable, such as parsnip or swede (rutabaga), if wished.

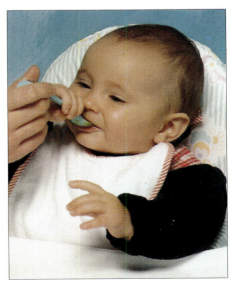

Lamb Hotpot

Makes: 600ml/1 pint/2½ cups

115g/4oz potato

115g/4oz carrot

115g/4oz swede (rutabaga)

50g/2oz leek

115g/4oz lamb fillet

300ml/½ pint/1¼ cup water

pinch of dried rosemary

1 Peel the potato, carrot and swede, then rinse and chop into small cubes. Halve the leek lengthways, rinse well and slice. Place all the vegetables in a pan.

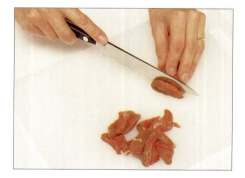

2 Rinse the lamb under cold water and chop into small pieces, discarding any fat.

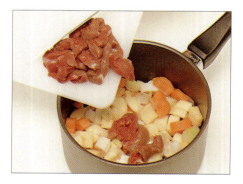

3 Add the meat to the pan with the water and rosemary. Bring to the boil, cover and simmer for 30 minutes or until the lamb is thoroughly cooked.

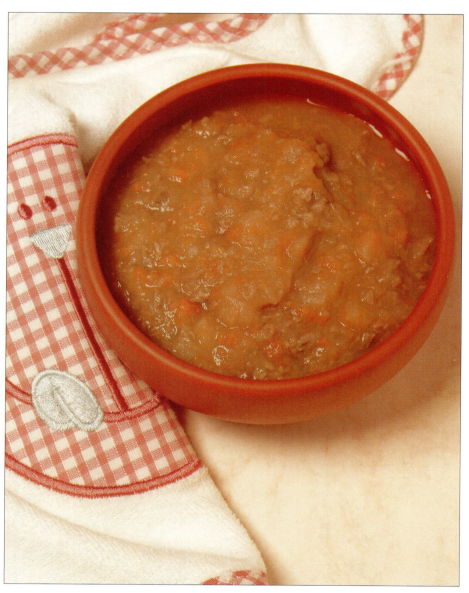

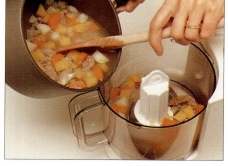

4 Process or mash the ingredients to the desired consistency.

5 Spoon a little into a bowl, test the temperature and cool if necessary, before giving to the baby.

6 Cover the remaining food and transfer to the refrigerator as soon as possible. Use within 24 hours.

• Suitable for freezing.

Lamb and Lentil Savoury

Makes: 600ml/1 pint/2½ cups

115g/4oz lamb fillet
115g/4oz swede (rutabaga)
1 celery stick
25g/1oz/2 tbsp red lentils
15ml/1 tbsp tomato ketchup
350ml/12fl oz/1½ cups water

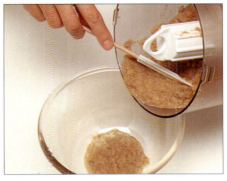

5 Cover the remaining food and transfer to the refrigerator as soon as possible. Use within 24 hours.

• Suitable for freezing.

4 Spoon a little into a bowl, test the temperature and cool if necessary, before giving to the baby.

VARIATION

Substitute green lentils or split peas for the red lentils and a small courgette (zucchini) for the celery stick.

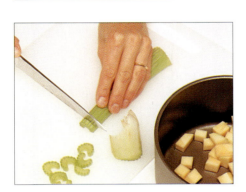

1 Rinse the lamb under cold water, trim off any fat and chop into small pieces. Peel the swede, place in a colander with the celery and rinse with cold water. Chop into cubes and place in a pan.

2 Put the lentils in a sieve (strainer) and rinse under cold water, picking out any black bits. Add to the pan with the lamb and ketchup.

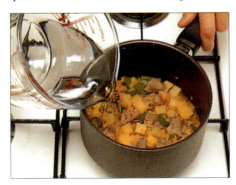

3 Add the water and bring to the boil, then cover and simmer for 40 minutes, or until the lentils are soft. Top up with extra water during cooking if necessary, then process or mash just enough to give the desired consistency.

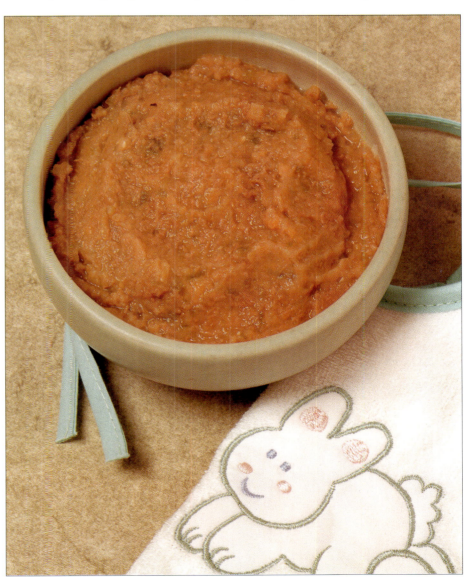

Country Pork and Runner Beans

Makes: 450ml/¾ pint/1⅞ cups

115g/4oz lean pork

115g/4oz potato

115g/4oz carrot

75g/3oz runner (green) beans

pinch of dried sage

350ml/12fl oz/1½ cups water

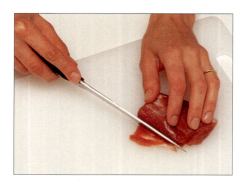

1 Rinse the pork under cold water, trim away any fat and gristle and chop into small cubes.

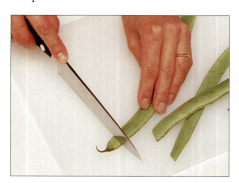

2 Peel the potato and carrot, trim the beans, rinse and chop.

3 Put the pork, potato and carrot in a pan with the sage and water. Bring to the boil, cover and simmer for 30 minutes.

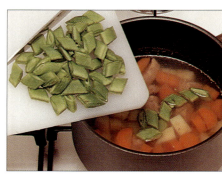

4 Add the beans and cook, covered, for a further 10 minutes, until all the vegetables are tender.

5 Process or mash to the desired consistency, then spoon a little into a bowl. Test the temperature before giving to the baby.

6 Cover and transfer the remaining food to the refrigerator. Use within 24 hours.

- Suitable for freezing.

VARIATION

Instead of the pork, use any lean meat in this recipe, such as chicken or turkey. Add broad (fava) beans, with the outer skin removed, in place of the runner beans.

TIPS

If runner beans are unavailable use French (green) beans, sugar snap peas or broccoli. Look out for ready-prepared diced pork in the supermarket. Cut into smaller pieces and be sure to remove any gristle before cooking.

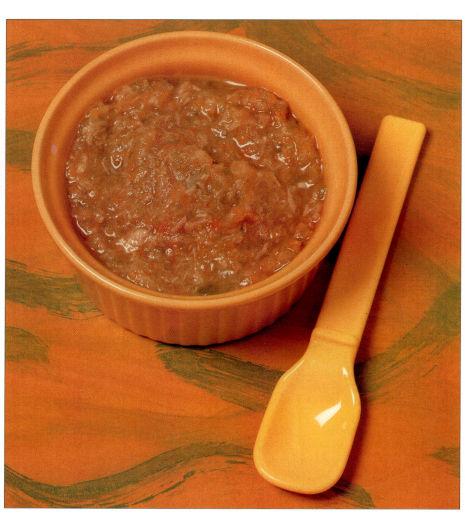

Pork and Apple Savoury

000Makes: 600ml/1 pint/2½ cups

175g/6oz lean pork
175g/6oz potato
175g/6oz swede (rutabaga) or parsnip
¼ onion
½ eating apple
300ml/½ pint/1¼ cups water
pinch of dried sage

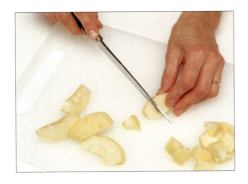

1 Preheat the oven to 180°C/ 350°F/Gas 4. Rinse the pork under cold water, trim away any fat and gristle, then chop. Peel and chop the vegetables. Peel, core and chop the apple.

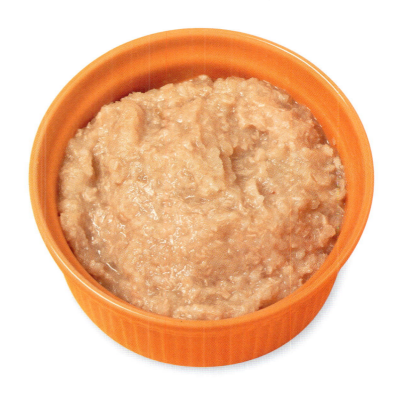

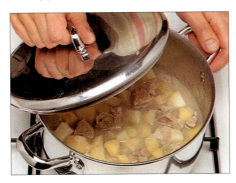

2 Put the meat, vegetables, apple, water and sage in a flameproof casserole, cover and bring to the boil, stirring once or twice.

3 Cover and cook in the oven for 1¼ hours, until the meat is tender, then process or mash to the desired consistency.

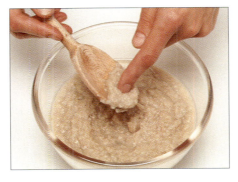

4 Spoon a little into a bowl, test the temperature and cool if necessary, before giving to the baby.

5 Cover the remaining food and transfer to the refrigerator as soon as possible. Use within 24 hours.

- Suitable for freezing.

TIP
The mixture can be cooked in a pan on the stove for 40 minutes, if preferred.

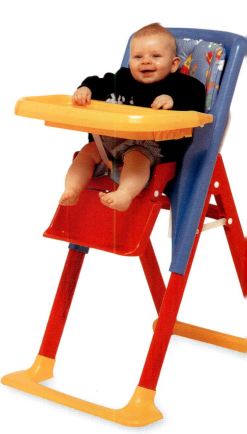

Nursery Kedgeree

Makes: 600ml/1 pint/2½ cups

50g/2oz/¼ cup long grain rice

25g/1oz/2 tbsp frozen peas

350ml/12fl oz/1½ cups formula milk

90g/3¼oz brick frozen skinless cod

2 hard-boiled egg yolks

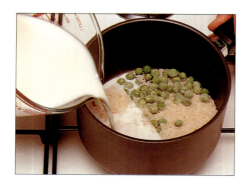

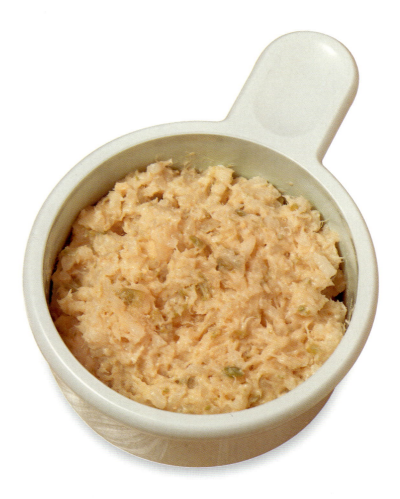

1 Place the rice, peas, milk and fish in a pan, bring to the boil, cover and simmer for 15 minutes, until the fish is cooked and the rice is soft.

2 Lift the fish out of the pan and break into pieces with a knife and fork, checking for bones.

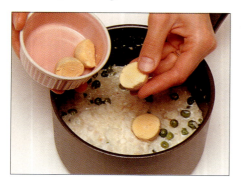

3 Stir the fish into the rice mixture and add the egg yolks.

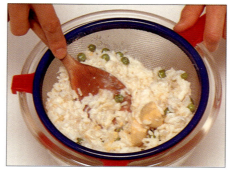

4 Mash with a fork to the desired consistency. Alternatively blend in a food processor or liquidizer, or press through a sieve (strainer).

5 Spoon a little into a bowl, test the temperature and cool if necessary, before giving to the baby.

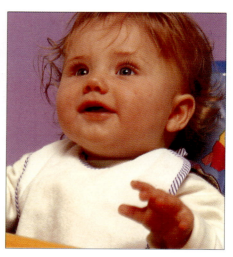

6 Cover the remaining kedgeree and transfer to the refrigerator as soon as possible. Use within 24 hours.

- Suitable for freezing.

TIP

Peas can be quite difficult to mash down. Check before giving to the baby as whole peas are difficult for her to chew.

Mediterranean Vegetables

Makes: 600ml/1 pint/2½ cups

3 tomatoes

175g/6oz courgettes (zucchini)

75g/3oz button (white) mushrooms

115g/4oz red (bell) pepper

20ml/4 tsp tomato ketchup

250ml/8fl oz/1 cup water

pinch of dried mixed herbs

40g/1½oz dried pasta shapes

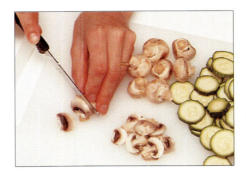

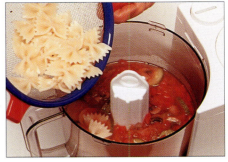

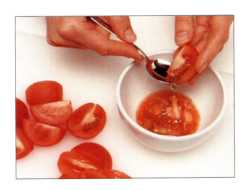

1 Make a cross cut in each tomato, put in a small bowl and cover with boiling water. Leave for 1 minute, then drain and peel off the skins. Cut into quarters and scoop out the seeds from the tomatoes.

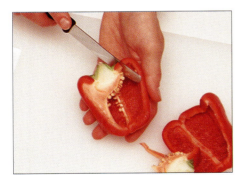

2 Trim the courgette and mushrooms and cut away the core and seeds from the pepper.

3 Rinse and slice the courgette and mushrooms. Chop the pepper.

4 Put the vegetables in a pan with the ketchup, water and herbs. Cover and simmer for 10 minutes, or until tender.

5 Meanwhile cook the pasta in boiling water for 8–10 minutes, until tender. Drain.

6 Mix the vegetables and pasta together and process or mash.

7 Spoon a little into a bowl, test the temperature and cool if necessary, before giving to the baby.

8 Cover remaining mixture and refrigerate. Use within 24 hours.

● Suitable for freezing.

TIP
For adventurous eaters add ½ clove crushed garlic at Step 3.

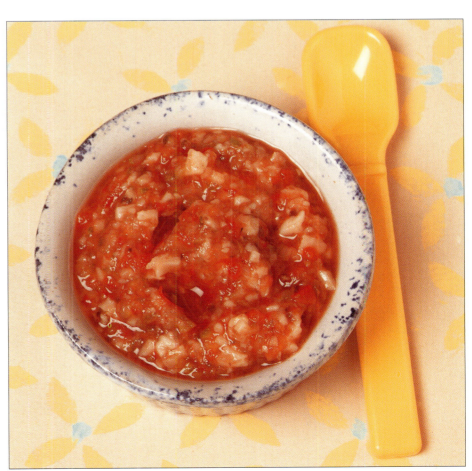

Pasta with Sauce

Makes: 600ml/1 pint/2½ cups

115g/4oz carrot
50g/2oz Brussels sprouts
25g/1oz green beans
25g/1oz/2 tbsp frozen corn
50g/2oz dried pasta shapes
350ml/12fl oz/1½ cups formula milk
50g/2oz Cheddar or mild cheese

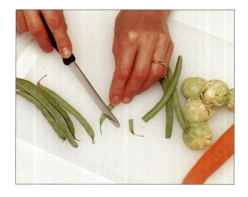

1 Peel the carrot, discard any discoloured outer leaves from the sprouts and trim the beans. Rinse and then chop into pieces.

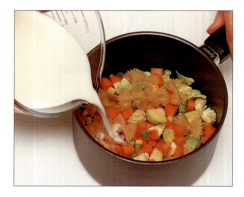

2 Place the prepared vegetables, corn, pasta and milk in a pan, bring to the boil and then simmer, uncovered, for 12–15 minutes, until the pasta is cooked.

TIP

Vary the vegetables depending on what you have in the refrigerator.

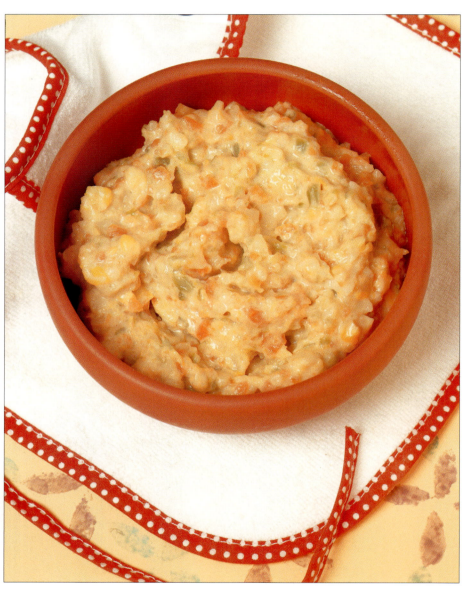

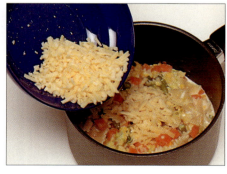

3 Grate the cheese and add to the vegetables, stirring until the cheese has completely melted.

4 Process or mash just enough to give the desired consistency, then spoon a little into a bowl. Test the temperature and cool if necessary, before giving to the baby.

5 Cover the remaining food and transfer to the refrigerator as soon as possible. Use within 24 hours.

● Suitable for freezing.

Apple and Orange Fool

Makes: 250ml/8fl oz/1 cup

2 eating apples

5ml/1 tsp grated orange rind and
   15ml/1 tbsp orange juice

15ml/1 tbsp custard powder

5ml/1 tsp caster (superfine) sugar

150ml/¼ pint/⅔ cup formula milk

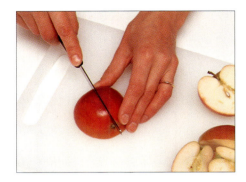

1 Quarter, core and peel the apples. Slice and place the apples in a pan with the orange rind and juice.

2 Cover and cook gently for 10 minutes, stirring occasionally until the apples are soft.

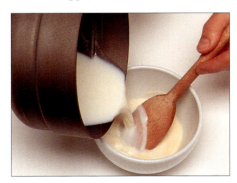

3 Blend the custard powder and sugar with a little of the milk to make a smooth paste. Bring the remaining milk to the boil and stir into the custard mixture.

4 Return the custard to the pan and slowly bring to the boil, stirring until thickened and smooth.

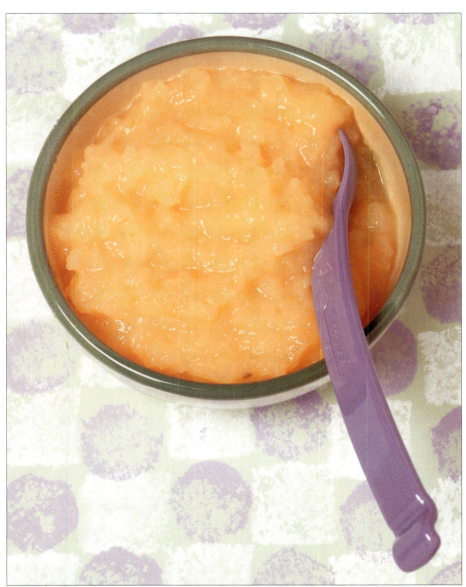

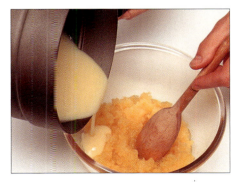

5 Process or mash the apple to the desired consistency. Add the custard and stir to mix.

6 Spoon a little into a bowl, test the temperature and cool if necessary, before giving to the baby.

7 Cover the remaining fool and transfer to the refrigerator as soon as possible. Use within 24 hours.

• Suitable for freezing.

Orchard Fruit Dessert

Makes: 450ml/³⁄₄ pint/1⁷⁄₈ cups

1 ripe pear

225g/8oz ripe plums

15ml/1 tbsp caster (superfine) sugar

15ml/1 tbsp custard powder

150ml/¼ pint/⅔ cup formula milk

1 Quarter, core, peel and slice the pear. Wash the plums, then cut in half, stone (pit) and slice.

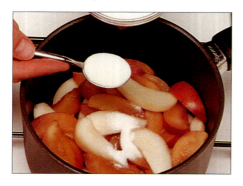

2 Put the fruit in a pan with 15ml/1 tbsp water and 10ml/ 2 tsp of the sugar. Cover and cook gently for 10 minutes, until soft.

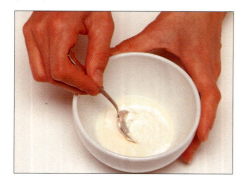

3 Blend the custard powder, remaining sugar and a little of the milk to make a smooth paste.

4 Bring the remaining milk to the boil and gradually stir into the custard mixture. Pour the custard back into the pan and bring to the boil, stirring, until it is both thickened and smooth.

5 Process or mash the fruit to the desired consistency and stir in the custard. Spoon a little into a bowl, test the temperature and cool if necessary, before giving to the baby.

6 Cover the remaining custard and transfer to the refrigerator as soon as possible. Use within 24 hours.

● Suitable for freezing.

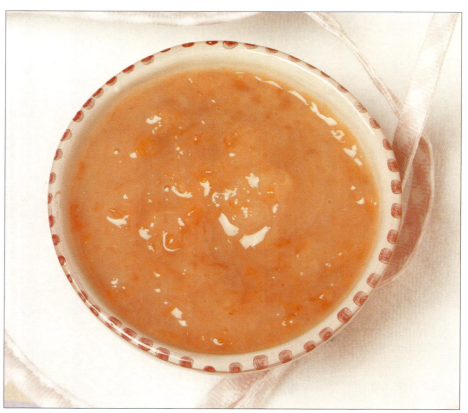

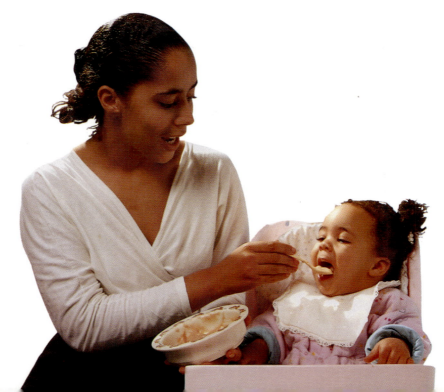

Peach Melba Dessert

Makes: 175ml/6fl oz/³⁄4 cup

1 ripe peach

25g/1oz fresh or frozen raspberries

15ml/1 tbsp icing (confectioners') sugar

115g/4oz Greek (US strained plain) yogurt

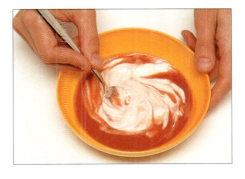

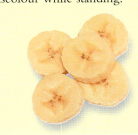

**VARIATION
Bananarama**
To make a single portion, use ½ a small banana and 15ml/1 tbsp of Greek (US strained plain) yogurt. Mash the banana until smooth and add the yogurt. Stir to mix and serve immediately. Do not make this dessert in advance, as the banana will discolour while standing.

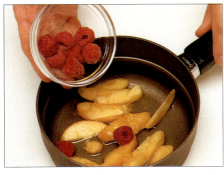

4 Set aside to cool, then stir in the sugar and swirl in the yogurt. Spoon a little into a baby dish.

5 Cover the remaining dessert and transfer to the refrigerator. Use within 24 hours.

1 Halve the peach, discard the stone (pit), then peel and slice. Place in a pan with the raspberries and 15ml/1 tbsp water.

2 Cover and cook gently for 10 minutes, until soft.

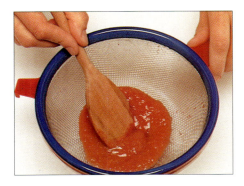

3 Purée and press through a sieve (strainer) to remove the raspberry pips (seeds).

TIP
The finished dessert is not suitable for freezing, but the sweetened fruit purée can be frozen in sections of an ice-cube tray. Defrost cubes of purée and mix each cube with 15ml/1 tbsp yogurt.

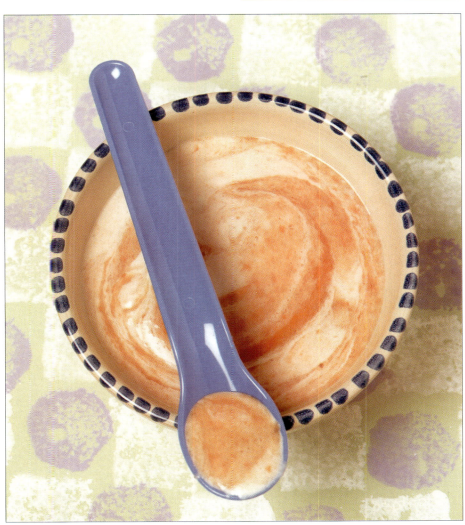

58

STAGE 4: NINE TO TWELVE MONTHS

GRADUALLY PROGRESS FROM MINCED TO CHOPPED OR ROUGHLY MASHED FOOD. BY NOW YOUR BABY WILL BE ABLE TO JOIN IN WITH FAMILY MEALS AND EAT A LITTLE OF WHAT YOU ARE EATING. ENSURE THAT YOUR BABY IS EATING THREE MAIN MEALS AND TWO TO THREE SNACK MEALS PER DAY. YOUNG CHILDREN DEVELOP AT AN INCREDIBLY FAST RATE AND SO NEED TO EAT LITTLE AND OFTEN TO SUSTAIN ENERGY AND GROWTH LEVELS. AGAIN, FOODS FROM THE PREVIOUS SECTIONS CAN STILL BE SERVED TO YOUR BABY; JUST ADJUST THE TEXTURES AS NECESSARY.

Suitable Foods

FOODS TO INCLUDE

- whole eggs
- finely ground nuts
- more flavourings – stock (bouillon) cubes if part of a family-size casserole
- greater selection of finger foods – slices of peeled fruit (such as dessert apple or pear), raw carrot and cucumber sticks, small squares of cooked chicken
- selection of foods from the four main food groups – carbohydrates (cereals, bread, potatoes, rice, pasta); fruit and vegetables; protein (meat, poultry, fish, eggs, beans, peas, lentils, tofu, nuts); milk and milk products (cheese, yogurt, butter).

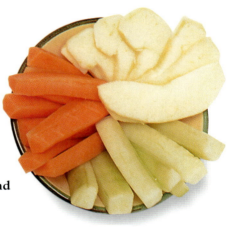

Apple, carrot and cucumber

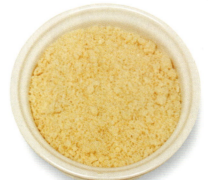

Ground nuts

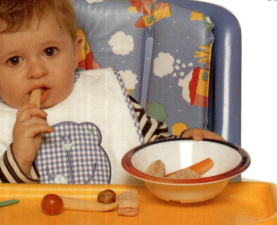

Whole egg

Left: *Finger foods – such as chopped raw vegetables and fruit pieces – come into their own at this age, and children love to help themselves.*

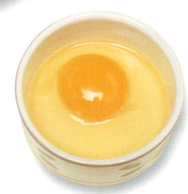

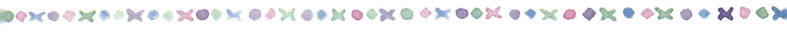

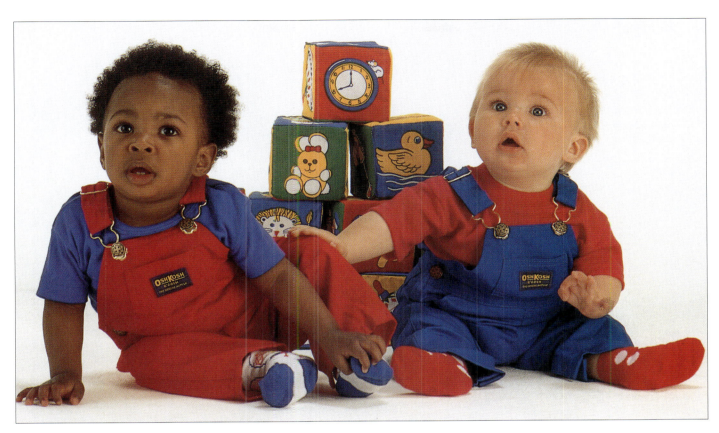

Above and below right: *Active children develop at a fast rate and need to eat little and often to sustain their energy levels.*

Below: *Though now a very small list, there are still some foods it is important to omit.*

FOODS TO AVOID
- keep salt to a minimum and omit if possible
- sugar: add just enough to make the food appetizing without being overly sweet
- honey
- fat: trim visible fat off raw meat, grill rather than fry
- organ meats – liver, kidney

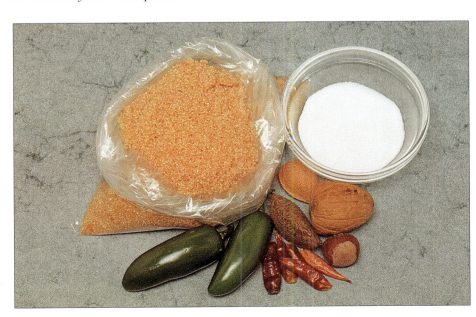

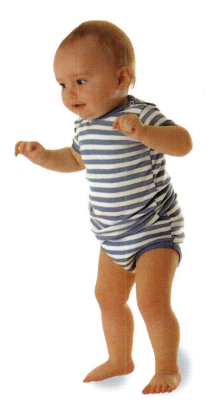

I Can Feed Myself!

Encouraging your baby to feed herself can be a truly messy business. Some babies are interested from a very early age, and those little fingers seem to move like lightning grabbing the bowl or the spoon you're using to feed them with. Give your baby a second spoon to play with, leaving you more able to spoon in the lunch.

As your baby grows, offer her a few finger foods to hold and hopefully eat, while you continue to feed from a spoon. Cooked carrot sticks, broccoli and cauliflower florets are soft on a young mouth and easy to chew. As your baby grows, you can introduce bread sticks and toast fingers.

Encourage your baby to pick up foods, and as her co-ordination improves and she gets the idea, more food will actually go where it is intended. Try to cut down on the mess by rolling up your baby's sleeves and covering clothes with a large bib, preferably with sleeves.

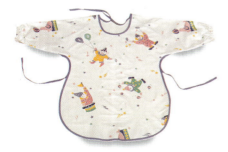

Above: *A bib with sleeves.*

Remove any hair bands and have a wet flannel at the ready.

Although it is tempting not to allow a baby to feed herself, try not to be frustrated by the mess. Babies that are encouraged to feed themselves will probably be more adventurous later on, and you will probably find there is less mess than with a baby who is always spoon fed

TEACHING YOUR BABY TO FEED HIMSELF

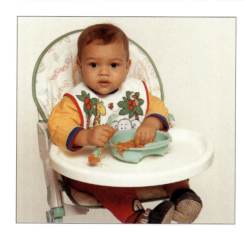

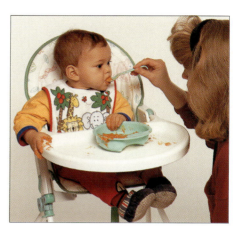

1 Cover your baby well – this can be very messy! Give him a spoon of his own to play with.

2 While you are feeding your baby, allow him to play with the food – with his hands or the spoon.

3 Let your baby use the cup and spoon by himself. Don't worry about spillage – there are bound to be lots of slips at this stage.

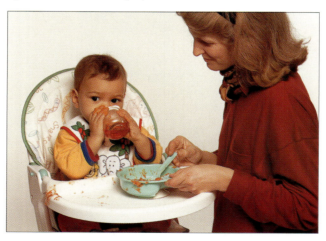

4 Keep tissues or a damp flannel available and clean as you go. Be patient and take things slowly.

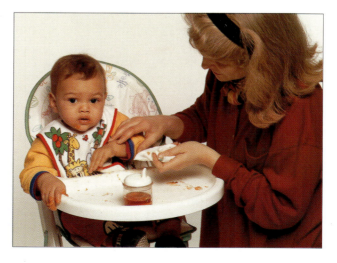

and keeps grabbing at the bowl. In addition, she will be able to join in your family meals and also give you the chance to eat your own meal before it gets cold.

WHAT TO DO IF YOUR CHILD CHOKES

● Don't waste time trying to remove food from your baby's mouth unless it can be done easily.
● Turn your baby, head down, supporting her head with your forearm and slap firmly between the shoulder blades.
● If this does not work, try again.
● Don't hesitate to ring your doctor or emergency services if worried.

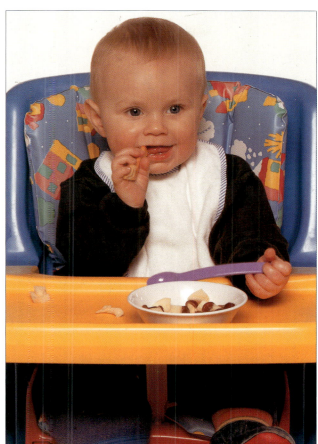

Left: *It is a real delight when your baby can begin to eat independently. Not only can you start to eat with your baby, and relax a little more, but he will also enjoy setting his own pace and eating his meal in the order he chooses. At this stage, the family can usually return to eating together around the table as a group.*

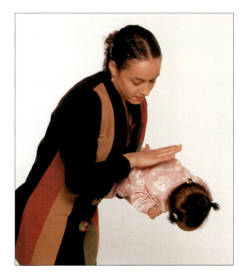

Above: *Don't be afraid to take quick, firm action in an emergency.*

COPING WITH THE MESS

As babies increase in size so too does the amount of mess they can create! It is quite incredible how just a few tablespoons of lunch can be spread across so many surfaces and so many items of clothing.
● Choose a large bib. Fabric bibs with a plastic liner are the most comfortable for babies to wear when tiny, moving on to a plastic pelican-style bib to catch food as they grow older. Check the back of your baby's neck as these can rub.

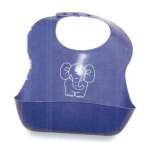

Above: *A hard plastic "pelican" bib.*

● If you plan to feed your baby in the dining room, then ensure you protect the carpet with an old sheet, pieces of newspaper, or a plastic tablecloth or groundsheet. It is vital to take this with you if visiting friends' houses.
● Give your baby a second spoon or small toy to play with so that she doesn't try to grab the laden spoon that you are holding.

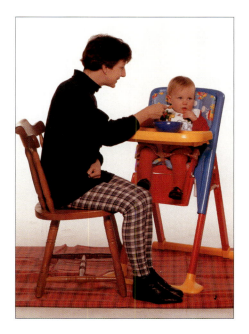

Above: *A plastic tablecloth or groundsheet on the floor will prevent carpet stains.*

FINGER FOODS

Finger foods are not only fun to eat
but help your baby's co-ordination.
Snacks play an important part in a
young child's diet as appetites may
be small, but energy and growth
needs are great. Choose foods that
are nutrient dense and avoid sweet
sugary snacks such as chocolate
biscuits (cookies).

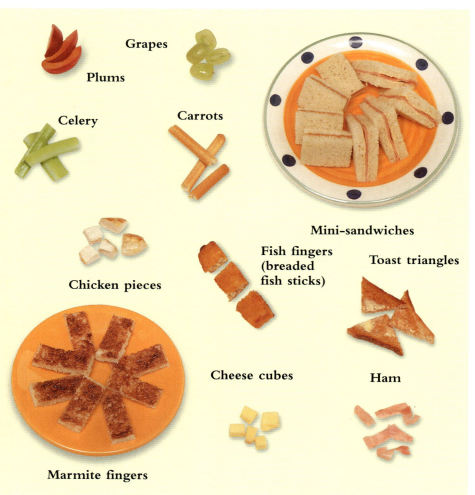

Grapes

Plums

Celery

Carrots

Mini-sandwiches

Fish fingers
(breaded
fish sticks)

Toast triangles

Chicken pieces

Cheese cubes

Ham

Marmite fingers

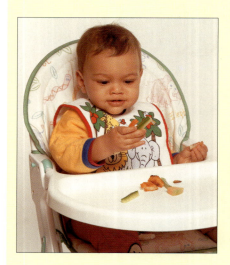

Above: *Your baby can eat at his own pace until he is full.*

TIPS

• Make sure the baby is comfortable
either on your lap or strapped into a
baby chair or high-chair.
• Check the temperature of the food
and make sure it is not too hot.
• Change the texture of the food:
some babies like quite wet mixtures,
some hate lumps, some like a few
lumps for interest, others prefer
food they can pick up – mini ham
sandwiches, thick slices of grilled
fish fingers (breaded fish sticks), even
picking up peas and corn.
• Encourage your baby to feed
herself; don't worry about the mess –
your baby is still learning – but
just mop up at the end.

• Try to keep calm. If your baby
keeps spitting food out, you may find
it less upsetting to offer bought food
rather than home-made so you don't
feel you've wasted time cooking.
• Try not to let your baby see you're
upset or annoyed. Even a one-year-
old can sense the power she can have
over you.
• If solid meals are well established,
give her a drink at the end of the
meal so that she is not full with
milk before she begins.
• Avoid biscuits (cookies) and sweet
things – your baby will soon learn that
if she makes a fuss when the savoury
is offered, dessert will soon follow.

• Remember no baby will starve
herself. Often babies who have been
good eaters become more difficult to
feed. Continue offering a variety
of food and don't despair.

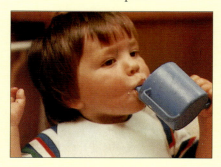

Above: *Give drinks at the end of the meal, or they will fill your baby up before he eats.*

Coping with a Fussy Eater

All children are fussy eaters at some stage. If meal-times are always calm and plates always clean, then your family must be one in a million. Even very young children learn the power they have over their parents, and meal-times give them a great opportunity to exercise it.

THE BABY SEEMS TO HAVE A SMALL APPETITE

Babies' appetites, like adults', vary enormously. Don't force feed your baby; if she's been eating well and then turns her head away or starts spitting out the food, it's a clear indication that she's had enough, even if the amount seems very small to you. Resist the temptation to encourage your baby to clear the dish: it is never helpful to force children of any age, and can be extremely counter-productive. Towards the end of the first year, a baby's weight gain usually slows down, and babies who have been good eaters become more difficult to feed. If you're worried, talk to your health visitor or doctor and regularly check your baby's weight.

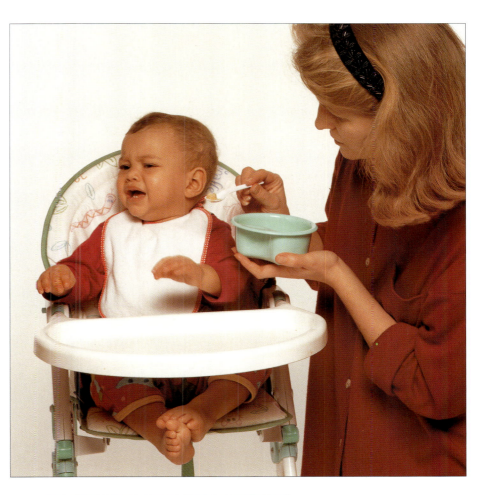

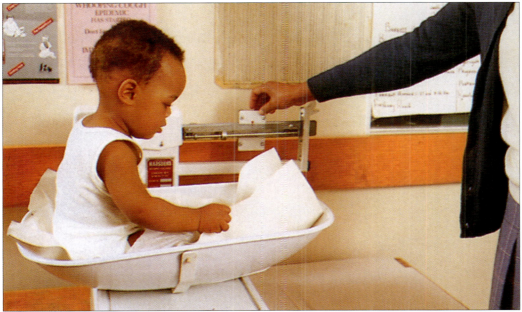

Above: *Don't worry when you encounter resistance in feeding: there never has been a baby that likes all foods, all the time.*

Left: *If you have any serious anxieties, see your doctor or health visitor and get your baby's weight checked regularly.*

The Importance of a Varied Diet

Once your baby progresses to more varied fruit and vegetable purées you are really beginning to lay down the foundations for a healthy eating pattern and sound nutritional habits that will take your baby through childhood and into adult life.

It is vitally important to include portions of food from each of the four main food groups – carbohydrates such as cereal, pasta and bread; fruit and vegetables; protein such as meat, fish and eggs; milk and milk products – every day. Don't forget to make sure that the types of food you choose are suitable for the age of your child.

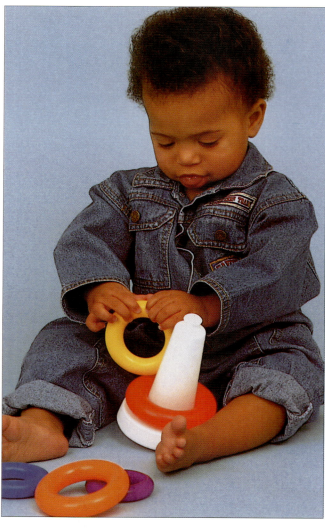

Left: Your baby is now at the age where the diet can and should be as diverse as any adult's. Variety is crucial for health reasons, and also has the benefit of allowing you many options for encouraging and maintaining the kind of interest in all types of food that will ensure good eating habits develop for the future.

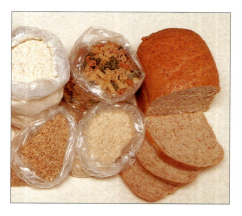

Group 1: *Cereals, bread, potatoes, rice and pasta.*

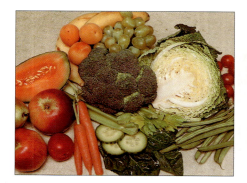

Group 2: *Fruit and vegetables* – bland tastes to start, such as potato, swede (rutabaga) and parsnip, then stronger flavours and a wider variety.

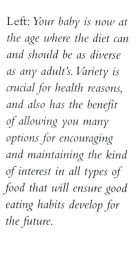

Group 3: *Meat and meat alternatives* – meat, poultry, fish, eggs, peas, beans, lentils, tofu, finely ground nuts.

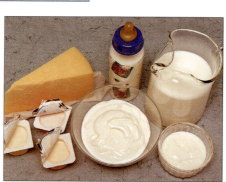

Group 4: *Milk and milk products* – milk, including soya milk, cheese, yogurt (plain at first, then flavoured).

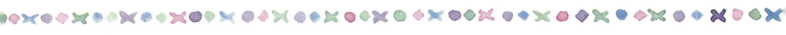

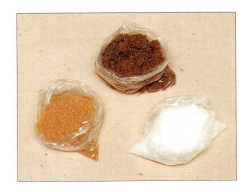

Group 5: *Sugars*

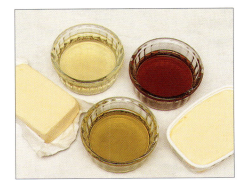

Group 6: *Fats and oils*

There are two more food groups that add palatability to the diet as well as contributing energy.

It is not recommended that you add sugar to baby foods or give lots of sugary drinks, particularly in the early days of weaning. Many of us have an inherent need for sweetness, but to cater to this without building in bad habits, try and include foods in the diet that are naturally sweet. Choose dessert apples instead of very sharp cooking apples, and mix bananas or ripe apricots with sharper-tasting fruits.

For those foods that are very sharp try to add 5ml/1tsp sugar per portion, so they become palatable without being overly sweet. Given the choice, your baby would prefer sweet flavours to savoury, so make sure you include a good range of tastes in the diet. Too much sugar or too many sweetened foods or drinks at this stage could lead to tooth decay

before the teeth are even through. Try to avoid offering biscuits (cookies) as a mid-morning or afternoon snack. Instead, encourage your baby to eat:

- a piece of banana
- a plain bread roll
- a few triangles of toast
- a milky drink
- a small container of yogurt

Watch the amounts of fat and oil you include in the diet. Avoid frying, especially when preparing first foods, as young babies have difficulty digesting such foods. As your baby develops, you can spread toast fingers with a little butter or margarine as easy-to-hold finger food. Maintain the milk feeds and introduce full-fat (whole) cow's milk after one year as the main drink of the day. Don't be tempted to serve skimmed (skim) milk, as the valuable fat-soluble vitamins A and D will be lost, and your baby may not get the energy needed for growth.

HOME-MADE OR MANUFACTURED FOODS?

Most parents use a combination of the two. Bought baby foods are convenient and often easier to use if going out for the day or until your baby's meals coincide with those of the rest of the family. Dried baby foods can be useful in the very early days, when your baby

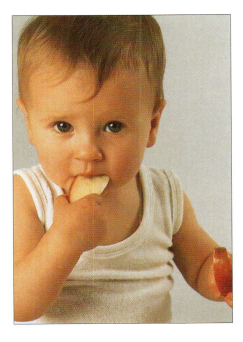

Above: *A piece of fruit or chopped vegetable is always preferable to a biscuit.*

is eating only a teaspoon of food at each meal. On the other hand, home-made foods can be batch-cooked or made with some of the ingredients from the main family meal and are often less trouble than you might expect. Added to this is the satisfaction of knowing your baby has eaten a wholesome meal and hopefully is acquiring a taste for home cooking.

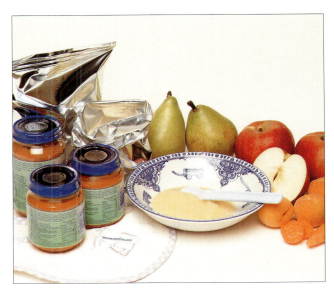

Left: *Home-made foods have the advantage that you know exactly what is in them. But there are some excellent products available for purchase that can save you time and effort and add hugely to your repertoire without any loss of dietary value.*

Lamb Couscous

Makes: 750ml/1¼ pint/3 cups

115g/4oz carrot

115g/4oz swede (rutabaga)

¼ onion

175g/6oz lamb fillet

5ml/1 tsp oil

10ml/2 tsp vegetable purée (paste)

30ml/2 tbsp currants or raisins

300ml/½ pint/1¼ cups water

50g/2oz couscous

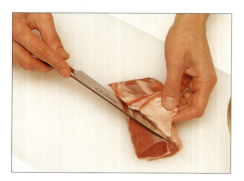

1 Peel the carrot, swede and onion, rinse and chop. Rinse the lamb, trim off any fat, and chop.

2 Heat the oil in a pan, and fry the lamb until browned.

3 Add the vegetables, cook for 2 minutes, then stir in the vegetable purée, currants and water. Cover and simmer for 25 minutes.

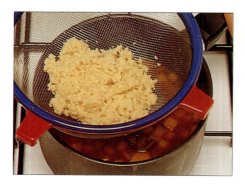

4 Put the couscous in a sieve (strainer) and rinse under cold running water. Cover and steam the couscous over the lamb pan, for 5 minutes.

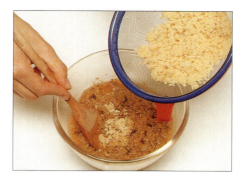

5 Chop or process the lamb mixture to the desired consistency. Fluff up the couscous with a fork and add to the lamb mixture stirring well.

6 Spoon a little into a bowl, test the temperature and cool if necessary, before giving to the baby.

7 Cover the remaining food and transfer to the refrigerator as soon as possible. Use within 24 hours.

● Suitable for freezing.

TIP
Look out for vegetable purée in tubes on the same shelf as the tomato purée in the supermarket.

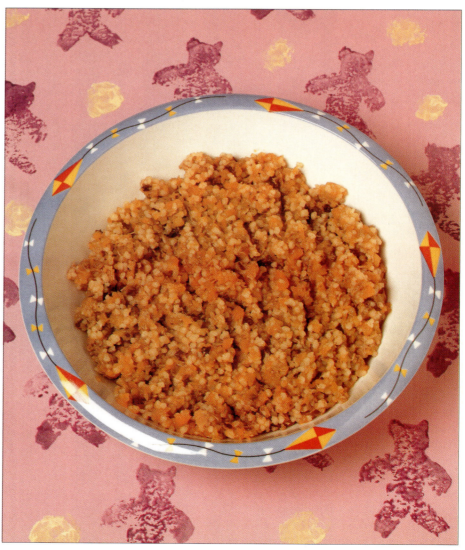

Paprika Pork

Makes: 600ml/1 pint/2½ cups

175g/6oz lean pork

75g/3oz carrot

175g/6oz potato

¼ onion

¼ red (bell) pepper

5ml/1tsp oil

2.5ml/½ tsp paprika

150g/5oz/⅔ cup baked beans

150ml/¼ pint/⅔ cup water

1 Preheat the oven to 180°C/ 350°F/Gas 4. Rinse the pork under cold water, pat dry and trim away any fat or gristle. Cut the pork into small cubes.

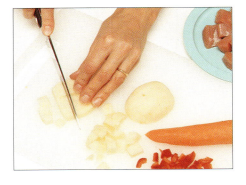

2 Peel the carrot, potato and onion. Cut away the core and remove any seeds from the pepper. Put into a colander, rinse under cold water, then chop into small pieces.

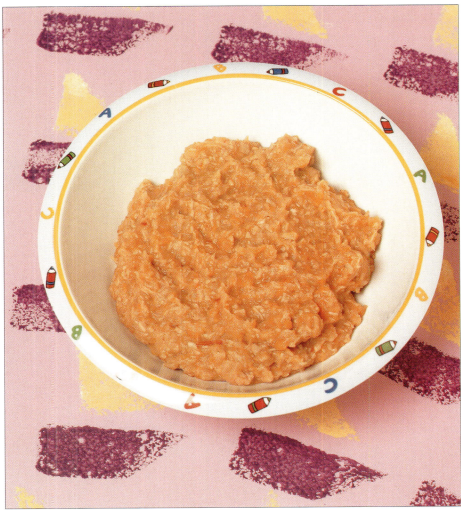

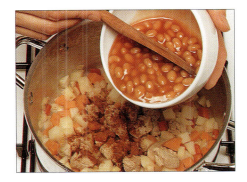

3 Heat the oil in a flameproof casserole, add the pork and fry for a few minutes, stirring until browned. Add the vegetables, cook for 2 minutes, then add the paprika, baked beans and water.

4 Bring back to the boil, then cover and cook in the oven for 1¼ hours, until the pork is tender.

5 Chop or process the casserole to the desired consistency, then spoon a little into a bowl. Test the temperature and cool if necessary, before giving to the baby.

6 Cover the remaining food and transfer to the refrigerator as soon as possible. Use within 24 hours.

● Suitable for freezing.

TIP

If using a food processor to chop the baby's dinner, drain off most of the liquid. Process, then stir in enough liquid for desired texture.

Chicken and Celery Supper

Makes: 600ml/1 pint/2½ cups

175g/6oz chicken thighs, skinned and boned
¼ onion
225g/8oz carrots
75g/3oz celery
5ml/1 tsp oil
10ml/2 tsp vegetable purée (paste)
250ml/8fl oz/1 cup water

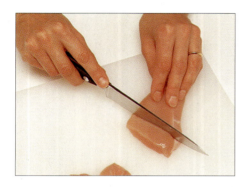

1 Rinse the chicken under cold water, pat dry, trim off any fat and cut into chunks.

2 Trim and rinse the vegetables and cut into small pieces.

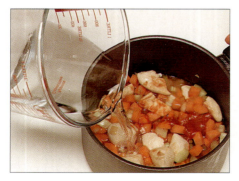

3 Heat the oil in a pan, add the chicken and onion, and fry for a few minutes, stirring until browned. Add the carrots, celery, vegetable purée and water. Bring to the boil, cover and simmer for 20 minutes, until tender.

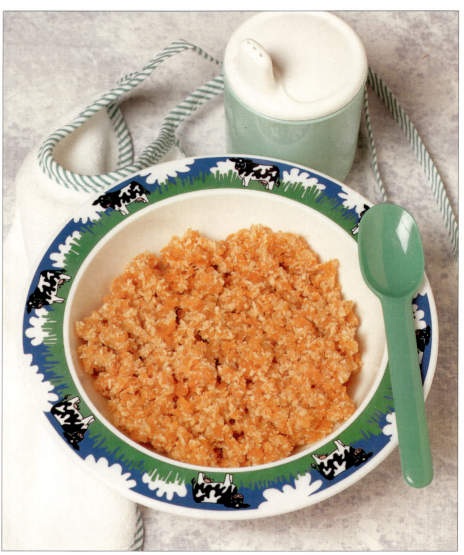

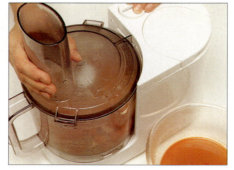

4 Chop or process the mixture to the desired consistency. If using a food processor, process the solids first and then add the liquid a little at a time.

5 Spoon a little into a bowl, test the temperature and cool if necessary, before giving to the baby.

6 Cover the remaining casserole and transfer to the refrigerator as soon as possible. Use within 24 hours.

• Suitable for freezing.

TIP
For extra flavour, add home-made stock instead of the water, or use commercial stock, but make sure it does not have a high sodium level.

Cauliflower and Broccoli with Cheese

Makes: 600ml/1 pint/2½ cups

175g/6oz cauliflower

175g/6oz broccoli

175g/6oz potato

300ml/½ pint/1¼ cups formula milk

75g/3oz Cheddar or mild cheese

1 Rinse the vegetables, then break the cauliflower and broccoli into florets. Slice the tender stems, but cut out and discard the woody core of the cauliflower. Peel and chop the potatoes into cubes.

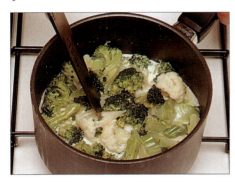

2 Place the vegetables and milk in a pan, bring to the boil, cover and simmer for 12–15 minutes, until quite tender.

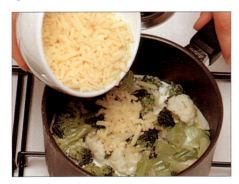

3 Grate the cheese and add to the vegetables, stirring until the cheese has melted.

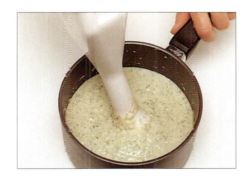

4 Process or mash the mixture to the desired consistency, adding a little extra milk if necessary.

5 Spoon a little into a bowl, test the temperature, and cool if necessary, before serving to the baby.

6 Cover the remaining food and transfer to the refrigerator as soon as possible. Use within 24 hours.

• Suitable for freezing.

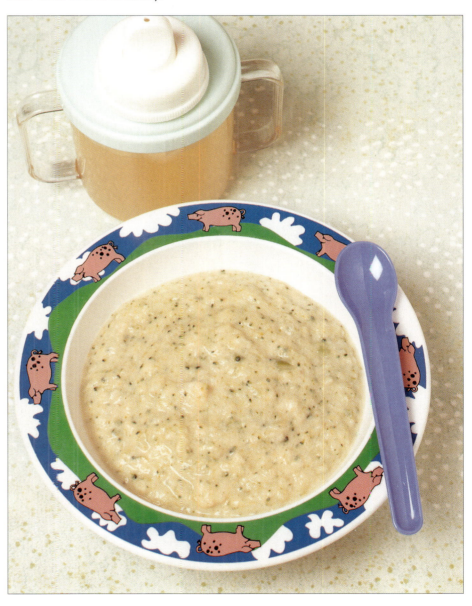

Tagliatelle and Cheese with Broccoli and Ham

Makes: 600ml/1 pint/2½ cups

115g/4oz broccoli

50g/2oz thinly sliced ham

50g/2oz Cheddar or mild cheese

300ml/½ pint/1¼ cups formula milk

50g/2oz tagliatelle

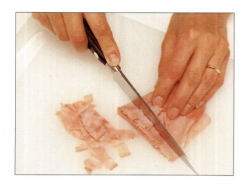

1 Rinse the broccoli and cut into small florets, chopping the stalks. Chop the ham and grate the Cheddar cheese.

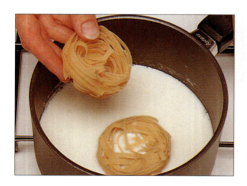

2 Pour the formula milk into a pan, bring to the boil and add the tagliatelle. Simmer uncovered for 5 minutes.

3 Add the broccoli and cook for 10 minutes, until tender.

TIP
Pasta swells on standing, so you may need to thin the cooled leftover mixture with extra formula milk before reheating.

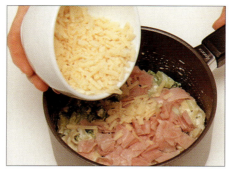

4 Add the ham and cheese to the broccoli and pasta, stirring until the cheese has melted.

5 Chop or process the mixture to the desired consistency and then spoon a little into a bowl. Test the temperature and cool if necessary, before giving to the baby.

6 Cover the remaining food and transfer to the refrigerator as soon as possible. Use within 24 hours.

- Suitable for freezing.

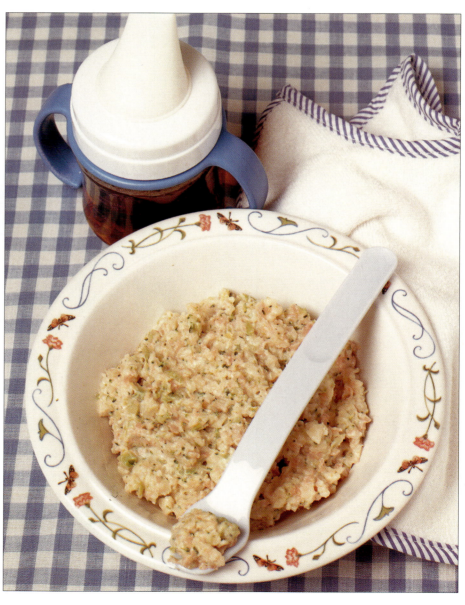

Baby Dahl

Makes: 600ml/1 pint/2½ cups

50g/2oz/¼ cup red lentils

¼ onion

2.5ml/½ tsp ground coriander

1.25ml/¼ tsp turmeric

350ml/12fl oz/1½ cups water

75g/3oz potato

75g/3oz carrot

75g/3oz cauliflower

75g/3oz green cabbage

1 Rinse the lentils under cold water, discarding any black bits.

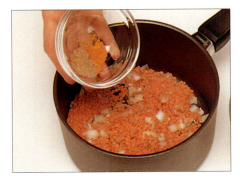

2 Chop the onion and add to a pan with the lentils, spices and water.

3 Bring to the boil, cover and simmer for 20 minutes.

4 Chop the potato, carrot and cabbage. Break the cauliflower into small florets.

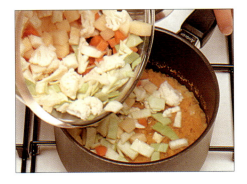

5 Stir the vegetables into the pan. Cook for 12–15 minutes.

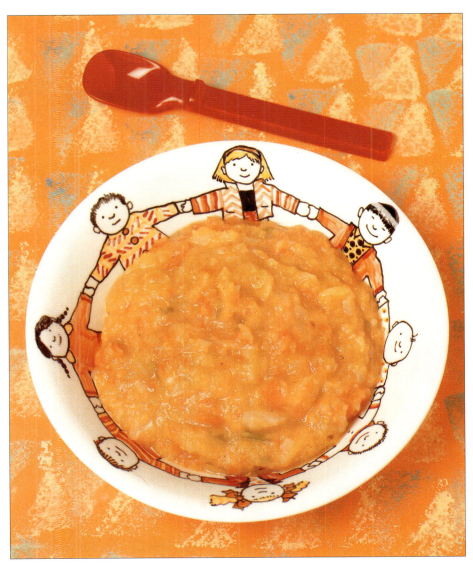

6 Chop or process the dahl to the desired consistency, adding a little extra boiled water if necessary.

7 Spoon a little dahl into a bowl, test the temperature and cool if necessary, before serving to the baby.

8 Cover the remaining dahl and transfer to the refrigerator as soon as possible. Use within 24 hours.

• Suitable for freezing.

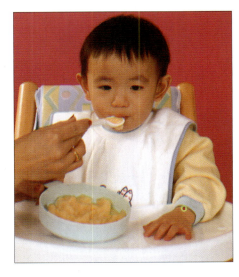

Fish and Cheese Pie

Makes: 450ml/¾ pint/1⅞ cups

225g/8oz potato

50g/2oz leek

50g/2oz button (white) mushrooms

90g/3½oz brick frozen skinless cod

250ml/8fl oz/1 cup formula milk

50g/2oz grated Cheddar,
  or mild cheese

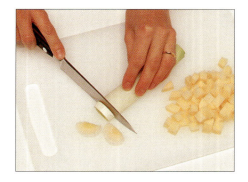

1 Peel the potato, halve the leek and trim the mushrooms. Place all the vegetables in a colander and rinse well with cold water, drain, then chop the vegetables.

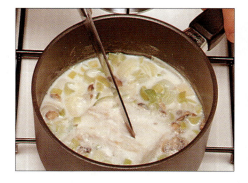

2 Place the vegetables in a pan with the frozen cod and milk. Bring to the boil, cover and simmer for 15 minutes, until the fish is cooked and the potatoes are tender when pierced with a knife.

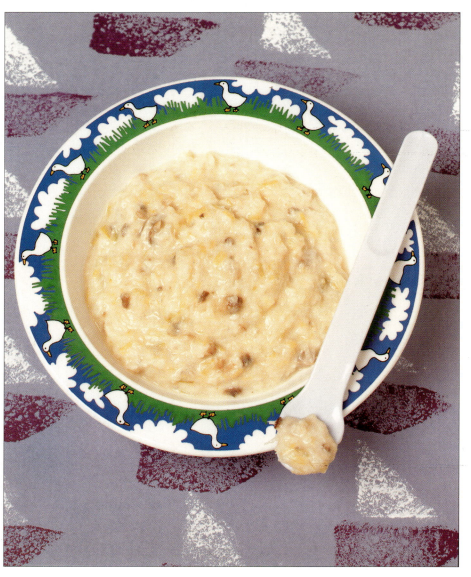

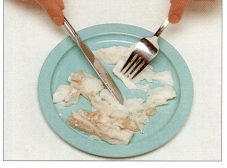

3 Lift the fish out of the pan with a slotted spoon and break into pieces with a knife and fork, checking carefully for bones.

4 Return the fish to the pan and stir in the grated cheese. Chop or process the mixture to give the desired consistency.

5 Spoon a little into a bowl, test the temperature and cool if necessary, before serving to the baby.

6 Cover the remaining fish pie and transfer to the refrigerator as soon as possible. Use within 24 hours.

● Suitable for freezing.

Fish Creole

Makes: 450ml/³⁄₄ pint/1⁷⁄₈ cups

50g/2oz celery

50g/2oz red (bell) pepper

300ml/½ pint/1¼ cups water

50g/2oz/¼ cup long grain rice

10ml/2 tsp tomato ketchup

90g/3½oz brick frozen skinless cod

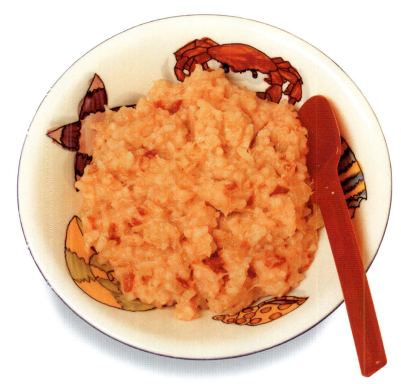

1 Trim the celery and discard the core and seeds from the pepper. Rinse and chop the vegetables.

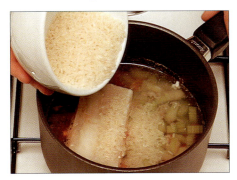

2 Bring the water to the boil in a pan and add the vegetables, rice, ketchup and cod.

3 Bring back to the boil, then reduce heat, cover and simmer for 15 minutes, until the rice is tender and the fish is cooked.

4 Lift the fish out of the pan with a slotted spoon. Use a knife and fork to check for bones.

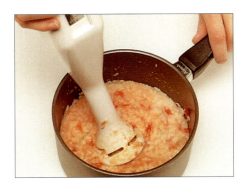

5 Stir the fish back into the pan and then chop or process.

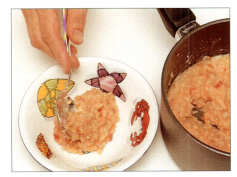

6 Spoon a little fish mixture into a small bowl, test the temperature and cool if necessary, before giving to the baby.

7 Cover the leftover fish creole and transfer to the refrigerator as soon as possible. Use within 24 hours.

• Suitable for freezing.

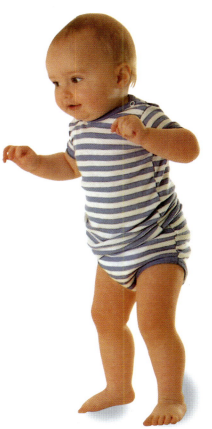

Chocolate Pots

Makes: 2

5ml/1 tsp cocoa

5ml/1 tsp caster (superfine) sugar

150ml/¼ pint/⅔ cup formula or
  cow's milk

1 egg

1 Preheat the oven to 180°C/
350°F/Gas 4. Blend the cocoa
and sugar with a little of the milk in a
small bowl to make a smooth paste.
Stir in the remaining milk and then
pour the mixture into a pan.

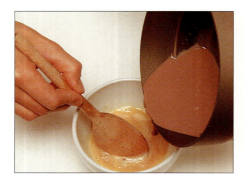

2 Bring just to the boil. Beat the
egg in a bowl, then gradually stir
in the hot milk, mixing well until the
mixture is smooth.

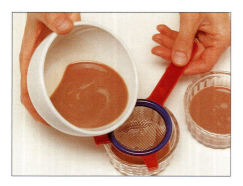

3 Strain the mixture into two
ramekin dishes to remove any
egg solids.

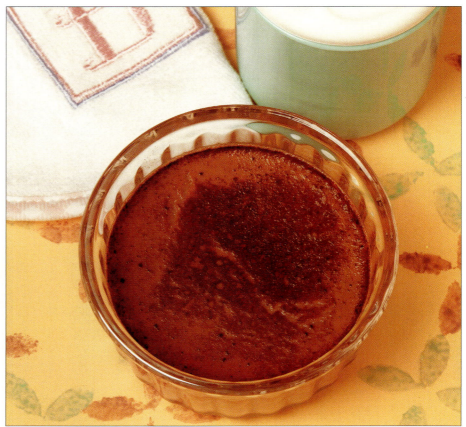

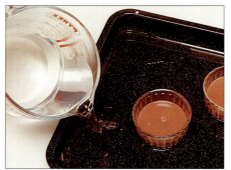

4 Place the dishes in a roasting pan
or shallow cake tin (pan). Pour
boiling water into the pan to come
halfway up the sides of the dishes.

5 Cook in the oven for 15–20
minutes, or until the custard has
set. Leave to cool.

6 Transfer to the refrigerator as soon
as possible. Serve one dessert and
use the second within 24 hours.

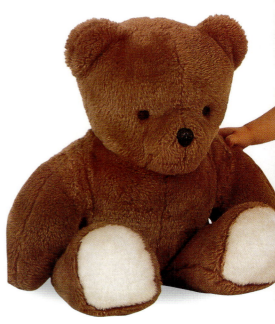

Vanilla Custards

Makes: 2

1 egg

5ml/1 tsp caster (superfine) sugar

few drops vanilla essence (extract)

150ml/¼ pint/⅔ cup formula or
  cow's milk

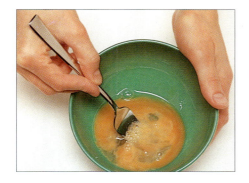

1 Preheat the oven to 180°C/
350°F/Gas 4. Using a fork, beat
the egg, sugar and vanilla essence
together in a bowl.

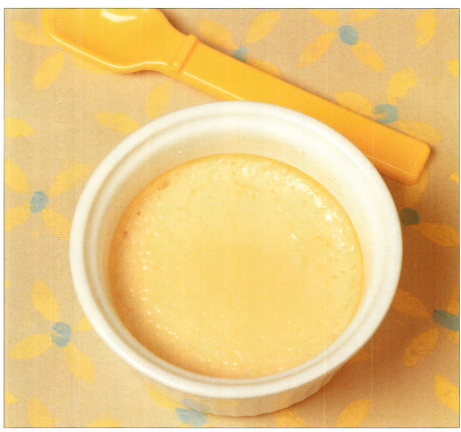

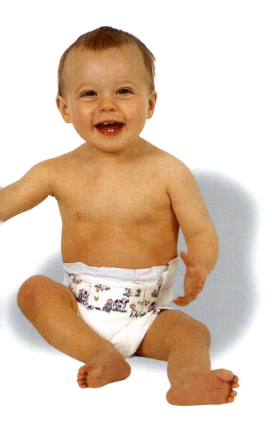

2 Pour the milk into a small pan
and heat until it is just on the
point of boiling.

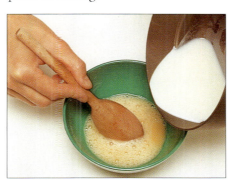

3 Gradually stir the milk into the
egg mixture, whisking or
beating until smooth.

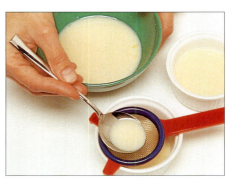

4 Strain into two ramekin dishes
and place in a roasting pan. Add
enough boiling water to come
halfway up the sides of the dishes.

5 Bake for 15–20 minutes, or until
the custard has set. Cool and
serve as for **Chocolate Pots.**

Marmite Bread Sticks

Makes: 36

little oil, for greasing

150g/5oz packet pizza base mix

flour, for dusting

5ml/1 tsp Marmite (yeast extract spread)

1 egg yolk

1 Brush two baking sheets with a little oil. Put the pizza mix in a bowl, add the quantity of water as directed on the package and mix to make a smooth dough.

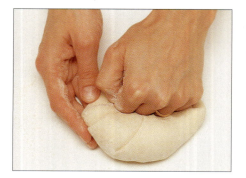

2 Knead on a lightly floured surface for 5 minutes, until smooth and elastic.

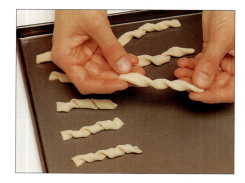

3 Roll out to a 23cm/9in square. Cut into strips 7.5cm × 1cm/3 × ½in, twisting each to give a corkscrew effect. Arrange on the baking sheets, slightly spaced apart.

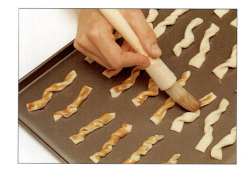

4 Mix the Marmite and egg yolk together and brush over the bread sticks. Loosely cover with oiled clear film (plastic wrap) and leave in a warm place for 20–30 minutes to rise.

5 Meanwhile preheat the oven to 220°C/425°F/Gas 7. Bake the bread sticks for 8–10 minutes, until well risen. Loosen but leave to cool on the baking sheet.

6 Serve one or two sticks to the baby. Store the rest in a plastic box for up to three days.

● Suitable for freezing up to three months in a plastic bag.

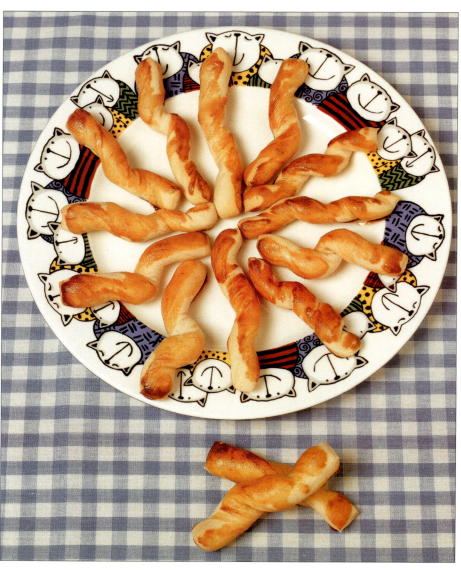

Bread Fingers with Egg

Makes: 16

2 slices bread

1 egg

30ml/2 tbsp formula or cow's milk

little butter and oil, for frying

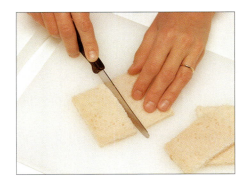

1 Trim the crusts off the bread, then cut each slice in half.

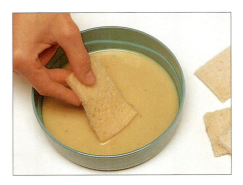

2 Beat the egg and milk in a shallow dish and dip the bread, one slice at a time, into the egg until coated on both sides.

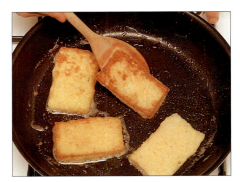

3 Heat a little butter and oil in a frying pan. Add the bread and fry until browned on both sides.

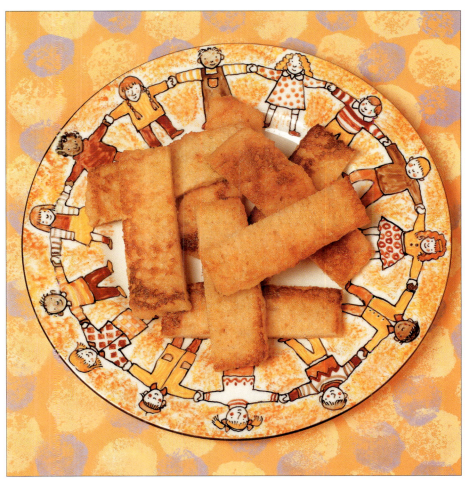

4 Cool slightly, cut into fingers and serve to the baby as finger food or as part of a meal.

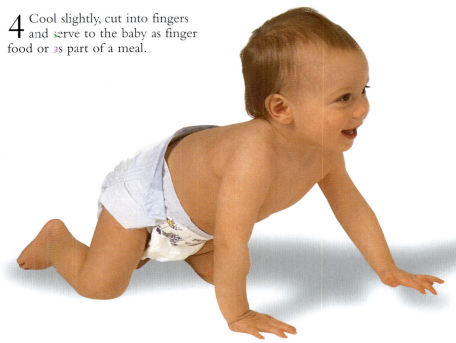

Cheese Straws

Makes: 42

little oil for greasing

175g/6oz/1½ cups plain (all-purpose) flour

75g/3oz/6 tbsp butter or margarine, cut into pieces

115g/4oz grated Cheddar or mild cheese

1 egg, beaten

1 Preheat the oven to 200°C/ 400°F/Gas 6. Brush two baking sheets lightly with oil.

2 Place the flour in a bowl, add the butter or margarine and rub in until the mixture resembles fine breadcrumbs. Stir in the grated cheese.

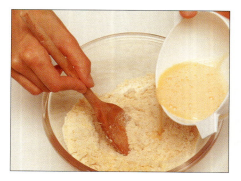

3 Reserve 15ml/1 tbsp beaten egg and then stir the rest into the pastry mixture. Mix to a smooth dough, adding water if necessary.

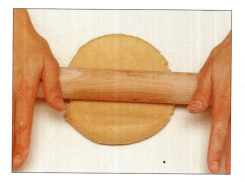

4 Knead lightly and roll out on a floured surface to a rectangle 30 × 20cm/12 × 8in. Brush with the remaining egg.

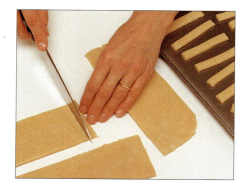

5 Cut into strips 7.5 × 1cm/ 3 × ½in and place on the baking sheets, spaced slightly apart.

6 Bake in the oven for 8–10 minutes, until golden brown. Loosen from but leave to cool on the baking sheets.

7 Serve one or two sticks to the baby and store the rest in a plastic box for up to 1 week.

• Suitable for freezing up to three months in a plastic box, interleaved with baking parchment.

TIP
Begin making these with mild cheese, and as your child gets more adventurous, change to stronger flavoured cheese.

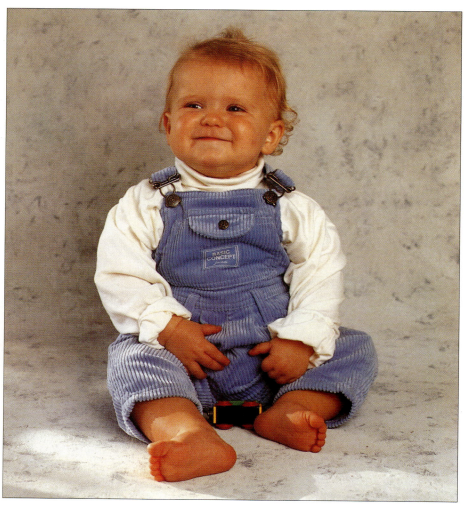

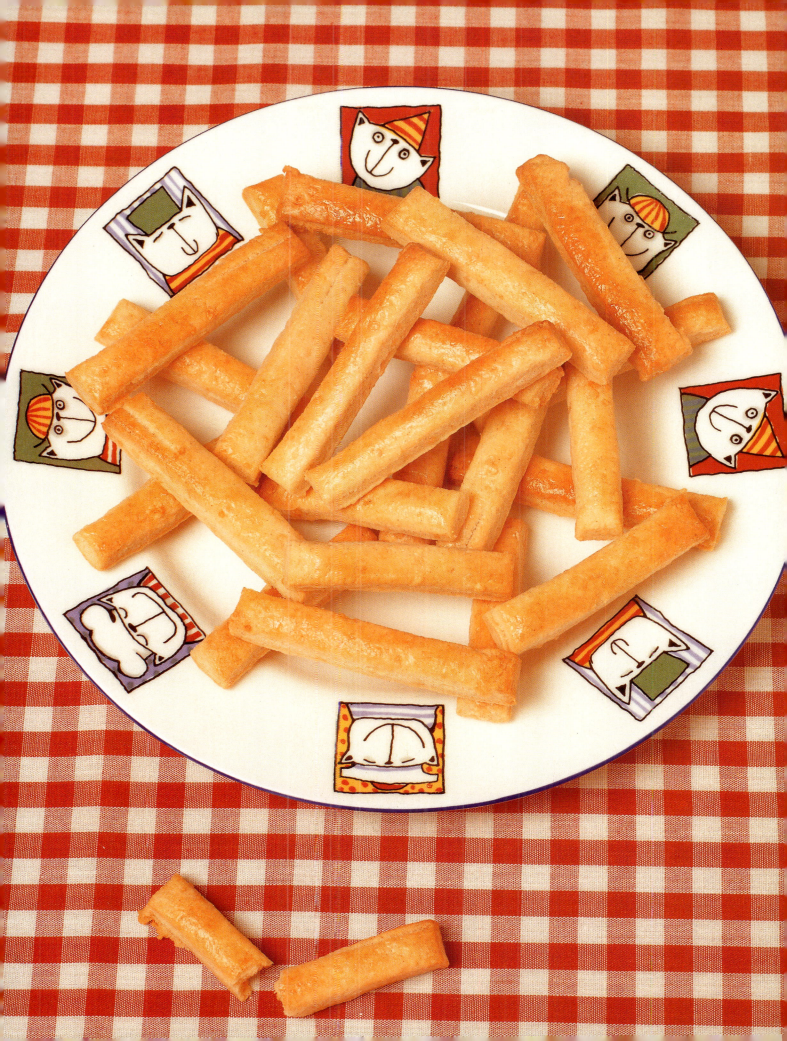

Mini Cup Cakes

Makes: 26

50g/2oz/4 tbsp soft margarine

50g/2oz/¼ cup caster (superfine) sugar

50g/2oz/⅓ cup self-raising (self-rising) flour

1 egg

1 Preheat the oven to 180°C/350°F/ Gas 4. Place 26 paper mini muffin cases on a large baking sheet.

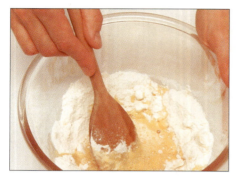

2 Put all the ingredients for the cake into a mixing bowl and beat together well until smooth.

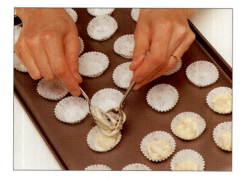

3 Divide the mixture among the cases and cook for 8–10 minutes, until well risen and golden.

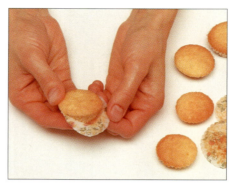

4 Transfer the cakes to a wire rack and leave to cool completely, then peel the paper off one or two cakes and serve to the baby.

5 Store the remaining cakes in a plastic box for up to three days.

● Suitable for freezing up to three months in a plastic box.

TIP
Cut a cup cake in half crossways and spread one half with a little sugar-free jam. Replace top half and serve to the baby.

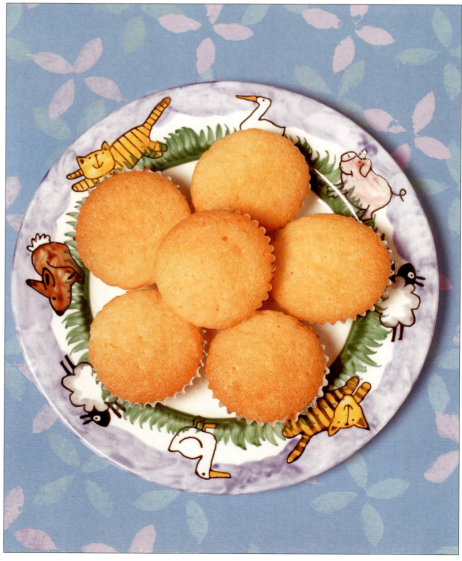

Shortbread Shapes

Makes: 60

little oil, for greasing

150g/5oz/1 cup plain (all-purpose) flour

25g/1oz/3 tbsp cornflour (cornstarch)

50g/2oz/¼ cup caster (superfine) sugar

115g/4oz/½ cup butter

extra sugar, for sprinkling (optional)

1 Preheat the oven to 180°C/350°F/Gas 4. Brush two baking sheets with a little oil.

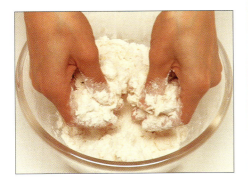

2 Put the flour, cornflour and sugar in a bowl. Cut the butter into pieces and rub into the flour until the mixture resembles fine breadcrumbs. Mould to a dough with your hands.

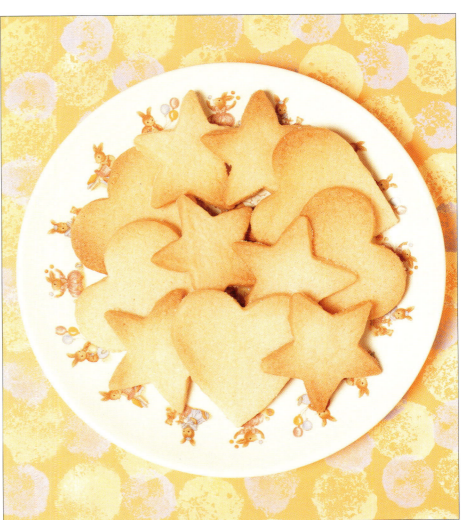

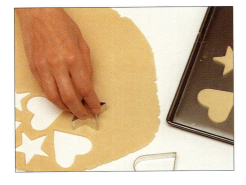

3 Knead lightly and roll out on a floured surface to a 5mm/¼in thickness. Stamp out shapes with small cookie or petits fours cutters.

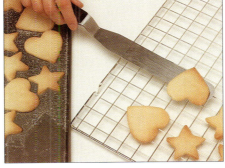

4 Transfer to the baking sheets, sprinkle with extra sugar, if liked, and cook for 10–12 minutes, until pale golden. Loosen with a knife and leave to cool on the baking sheets, then transfer to a wire rack.

5 Offer the baby one or two shapes and store the rest in a plastic box for up to one week.

TIP
These biscuits (cookies) will keep well in the freezer for three months. Pack in rigid plastic boxes and thaw in a single layer. If you prefer, you can freeze them before baking. Wrap well to prevent them taking up flavours from other food.

STAGE 5: FROM BABY TO TODDLER

Once your child has reached 12 months he or she will be enjoying a varied diet, and eating habits and personal food preferences will be developing. It is now vital to lay the foundations of a good and well-balanced eating regime. This is a time when food fads may also develop. Try to weather this period of fussy eating – all children experience it at some time. Even good eaters may go through a stage where eating habits vary significantly from day to day. Be guided by your child and try to think in terms of what the child has eaten over several days rather than worrying about what they don't eat on a particular day. The fad should go as quickly as it came, but while it lasts, meal-times will require extra patience.

Suitable Foods

Give your child a selection of foods in the four main food groups daily:

Cereal and filler foods: include three to four helpings of the following per day – breakfast cereals, bread, pasta, potatoes, rice.

Fruit and vegetables: try to have three or four helpings per day. Choose from fresh, canned, frozen or dried.

Meat and/or alternatives: one to two portions per day – meat (all kinds, including burgers and sausages), poultry, fish (fresh, canned or frozen), eggs (well cooked), lentils, peas and beans (for example chickpeas baked beans, red kidney beans), finely chopped nuts, smooth peanut butter, seeds, tofu, and Quorn.

Dairy foods: include 600ml/1 pint of milk per day or a mix of milk, cheese, and yogurt. For a child who stops drinking milk, use alternative ways of ensuring they get milk: try flavouring it or using it in custards, ice cream, rice pudding or cheese sauce. A carton of yogurt or 40g/1½oz of cheese have the same amount of calcium as 190ml/⅓ pint of milk.

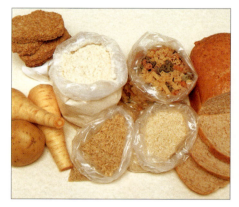

Above: *Cereal and filler foods, such as bread, pasta and rice.*

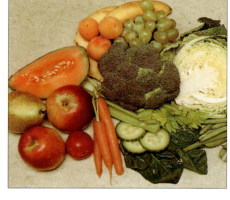

Above: *Fruit and vegetables, including frozen, dried and canned goods.*

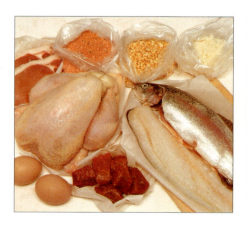

Above: *Meat and meat alternatives, such as beans, peas, lentils and nuts.*

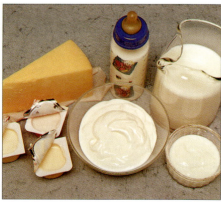

Above: *Dairy foods such as milk, cheese and yogurt.*

FATS

As adults we are all aware of the need to cut down on our fat consumption, but when eating together as a family, bear in mind that fat is a useful source of energy in a child's diet. The energy from fat is in concentrated form, so that your child can take in the calories she needs for growth and development before her stomach becomes overfull. Fat in food is also a valuable source of the fat-soluble vitamins, A, D, E and K, as well as essential fatty acids that the body cannot make by itself.

In general, fat is best provided by foods that contain not just fat but other essential nutrients as well, such as dairy products, eggs, meat and fish. Full-fat (whole) milk and its products such as cheese and yogurt, and eggs contain the fat-soluble vitamins A and D, while sunflower (sunflower-seed) oil, nuts and oily fish are a good source of various essential fatty acids.

It is wise to cut down on deep frying and to grill (broil) or oven bake foods where possible. All children love crisps (potato chips), but keep them as a treat rather than a daily snack.

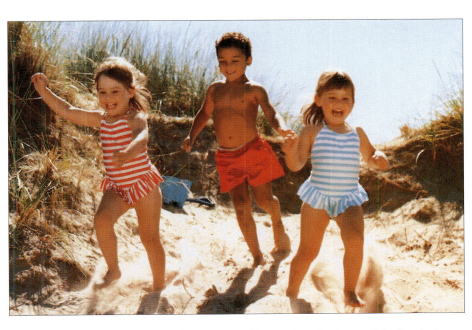

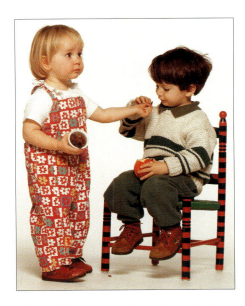

Above: *Keep sweets and chocolate as treats — give fruit and vegetables as snacks.*

FRUIT AND VEGETABLES

Fresh fruit and vegetables play an essential part in a balanced diet. Offer fresh fruit, such as slices of apple or banana, for breakfast and the evening meal, and perhaps thin sticks of raw carrot and celery for lunch. Instead of biscuits (cookies), offer your child raisins, apricots, satsumas, carrots or apple slices if she wants a mid-morning or afternoon snack. Keep the fruit bowl within easy reach so she may be tempted to pick up a banana as she walks through the kitchen.

Above: *A good mixture of the four basic food types will provide maximum energy and vitality for growing children.*

SNACKS

Young children cannot eat enough food at meal-times to meet their requirements for energy and growth, and snacks can play a vital part in meeting these needs. However, keep biscuits and crisps as a treat. They contain little goodness and are bad for the teeth. At meal-times keep sweets (candy) out of sight until the main course has been eaten.

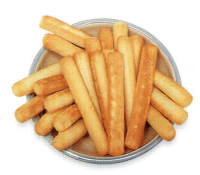

Bread sticks

Raisins

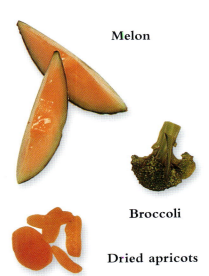

Melon

Broccoli

Dried apricots

Coping With a Fussy Eater

We all have different sized appetites whatever our age, and young children are no exception. Children's appetites fluctuate greatly and often tail off just before a growth spurt. All children go through food fads; some just seem to last longer and be more difficult than others.

A toddler's appetite varies enormously, and you may find that she will eat very well one day and eat hardly anything the next. Be guided by your toddler, and try to think in terms of what the child has eaten over several days rather than just concentrating on one day.

At the time, it can be very frustrating and worrying. Try not to think of the food that you have just thrown away, but try to think more in the long term. Jot down the foods that your child has actually eaten over three or four days, or up to a week. You may actually be surprised that it isn't just yogurts and crisps after all!

Once you have a list, you may find a link between the foods your child eats and the time of day. Perhaps your child eats better when eating with the family, or when the house is quiet. If you do find a link, then build on it. You might find that your child is snacking on chocolate, doughnuts or soft drinks when out with friends, and that fussiness at home is really a full tummy. Or it may be that by cutting out a milk drink and a biscuit (cookie) mid-morning and offering a sliced apple instead, your child may not be so full at lunchtime. Perhaps you could hide the biscuit tin (cookie jar) once visitors have had one, so that tiny hands can't keep reaching for more.

If your toddler seems hungrier at breakfast, then you could offer French toast, a grilled sausage or a few banana slices with her cereal.

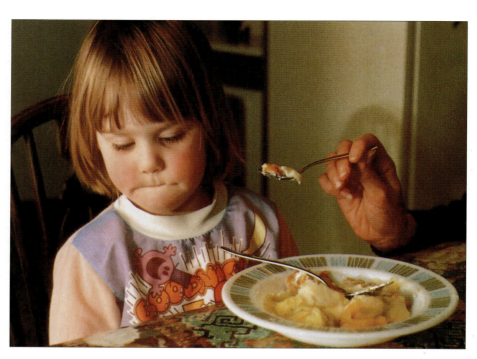

Above: *Don't panic about food rejection. Be patient and keep a journal listing what your child actually does eat.*

Right: *Fresh, healthy snacks of fruit, such as apples, will preserve your child's appetite for main meals.*

Although this may all sound very obvious, when rushing about caring for a toddler and perhaps an older child or new baby as well, life can become rather blurred, and it can be difficult to stand back and look at things objectively.

REFUSING TO EAT

A child will always eat if she is hungry, although it may not be when you want her to eat. A child can stay fit and healthy on surprisingly little. Providing your child is growing and gaining weight, then don't fuss, but if you are worried, talk to your doctor or health visitor. Take the lead from your child, never force feed a child and try not to let meal-times become a battleground.

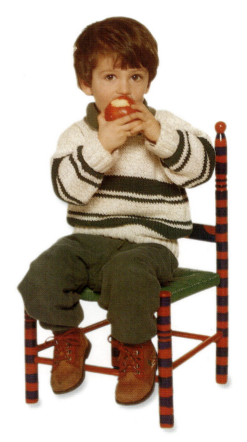

MAKING MEAL-TIMES FUN

Coping with a fussy eater can be incredibly frustrating. The less she eats, the crosser you get, and so the spiral goes on as your toddler learns how to control meal-times. To break this vicious circle, try diffusing things by involving your child in the preparation of the meal. You could pack up a picnic with your child's help, choosing together what to take. Then go somewhere different to eat – it could be the back garden, the swings or even the car. Alternatively, have a dollies' or teddies' tea party or make a camp under the dining table or even in the cupboard under the stairs.

Even very young children enjoy having friends round for tea. If your child is going through a fussy or non-eating stage, invite over a little friend with a good appetite. Try to take a back seat, and don't make a fuss over how much the visiting child eats compared to your own.

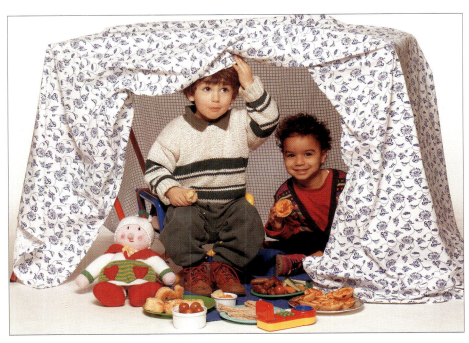

Above: *Changing the scene and breaking routine can help greatly.*

Below: *Making the meal a special event can distract the child from any eating worries.*

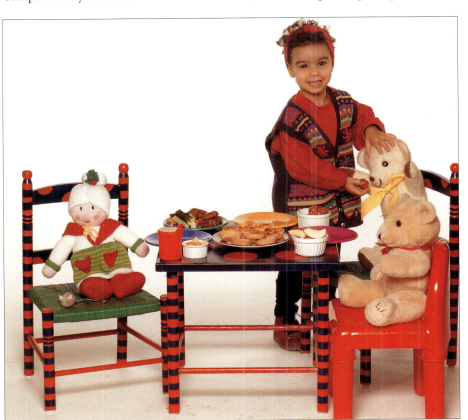

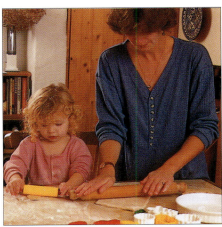

Above: *Getting your child to help you cook the food will encourage her to eat it, too.*

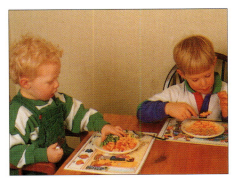

Above: *Children are more likely to eat with friends of their own age around them.*

Shepherd's Pie

Serves 2

½ small onion

175g/6oz lean minced (ground) beef

10ml/2 tsp plain (all-purpose) flour

30ml/2 tbsp tomato ketchup

150ml/¼ pint/⅔ cup beef stock

pinch of mixed herbs

50g/2oz swede (rutabaga)

½ small parsnip, about 50g/2oz

1 medium potato, about 115g/4oz

10ml/2 tsp milk

15g/½oz/1 tbsp butter or margarine

½ carrot

40g/1½oz/3 tbsp frozen peas

salt and pepper (optional)

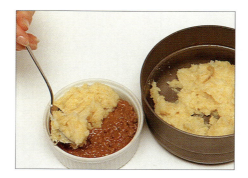

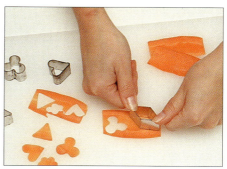

5 Spoon the meat into two 250ml/8fl oz/1 cup ovenproof dishes. Place the mashed vegetables on top, fluffing them up with a fork. Dot with butter or margarine.

6 Place both the pies on a baking sheet and cook for 25–30 minutes, until browned on top and bubbly.

7 Peel and thinly slice the carrot lengthways. Stamp out shapes with petits fours cutters. Cook in a pan of boiling water with the peas for 5 minutes. Drain and serve with the shepherd's pies. Remember that baked pies are very hot when they come out of the oven. Always allow to cool slightly before serving to children.

1 Preheat oven to 190°C/375°F/ Gas 5. Finely chop the onion, and place in a small pan with the mince and dry fry over a low heat, stirring, until the mince is evenly browned.

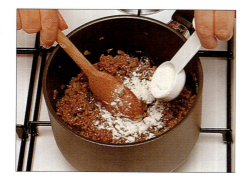

2 Add the flour, stirring, then add the ketchup, stock, mixed herbs and seasoning, if liked. Bring to the boil, cover the pan and simmer gently for approximately 30 minutes, stirring occasionally.

3 Meanwhile, chop the swede, parsnip and potato, and cook for 20 minutes, until tender. Drain.

4 Mash with the milk and half of the butter or margarine.

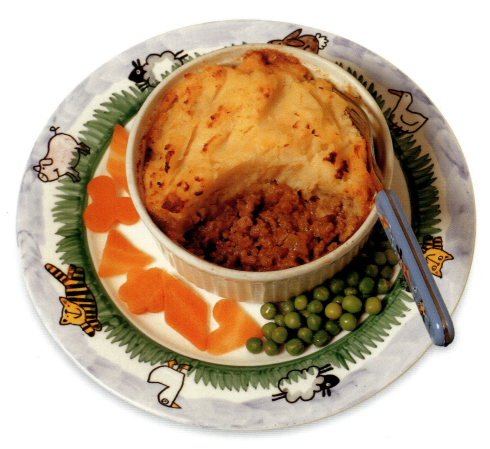

Lamb Stew

Serves 2

115g/4oz lamb fillet
¼ small onion
1 small carrot, about 50g/2oz
½ small parsnip, about 50g/2oz
1 small potato
5ml/1 tsp oil
150ml/¼ pint/⅔ cup lamb stock
pinch of dried rosemary
salt and pepper (optional)
crusty bread, to serve

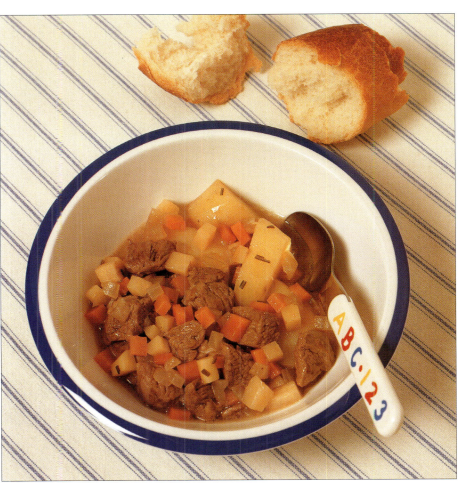

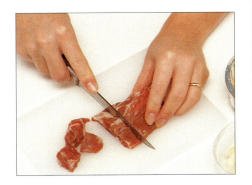

1 Rinse the lamb under cold water and pat dry. Cut away any fat from the meat and cut into small cubes. Finely chop the onion, then dice the carrot and parsnip and cut the potato into slightly larger pieces.

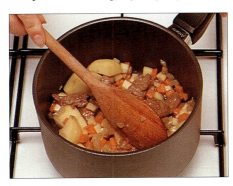

2 Heat the oil in a medium-size pan, add the lamb and onion, and fry gently until browned. Add the carrot, parsnip and potato, and fry the lamb and vegetables for a further 3 minutes, stirring.

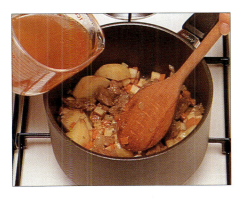

3 Add the lamb stock, dried rosemary and a little salt and pepper, if liked. Bring to the boil, cover and simmer for 35–40 minutes, or until the meat is tender and moist.

4 Spoon the stew into shallow bowls and cool slightly before serving with crusty bread.

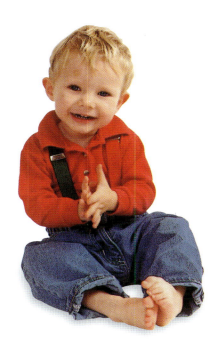

Fish and Cheese Pies

Serves 2

1 medium potato, about 150g/5oz

25g/1oz green cabbage

115g/4oz cod or hoki fillets

25g/1oz/2 tbsp frozen corn

150ml/¼ pint/⅔ cup milk

15ml/1 tbsp butter or margarine

15ml/1 tbsp plain (all-purpose) flour

25g/1oz/¼ cup grated Red Leicester or mild cheese

5ml/1 tsp sesame seeds

carrots and mangetouts (snowpeas), to serve

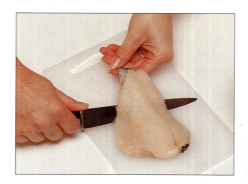

1 Peel and cut the potato into chunks and shred the cabbage. Cut any skin away from the fish fillets and rinse under cold water.

2 Bring a pan of water to the boil, add the potato and cook for 10 minutes. Add the cabbage and cook for a further 5 minutes until tender. Drain.

3 Meanwhile, place the fish fillets, the corn and all but 10ml/2 tsp of the milk in a second pan. Bring to the boil, then cover the pan and simmer very gently for 8–10 minutes, until the fish flakes easily when pressed with a knife.

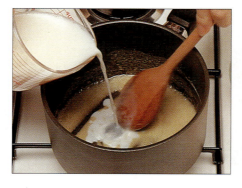

4 Strain the fish and corn, reserving the cooking liquid. Wash the pan, then melt the butter or margarine in the pan. Stir in the flour, then gradually add the reserved cooking liquid and bring to the boil, stirring until thickened and smooth.

5 Add the fish and corn with half of the grated cheese. Spoon into two small ovenproof dishes.

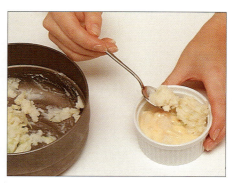

6 Mash the potato and cabbage with the remaining 10ml/2 tsp milk. Stir in half of the remaining cheese and spoon the mixture over the fish. Sprinkle with the sesame seeds and the remaining cheese.

7 Cook under a preheated grill until the topping is browned. Cool slightly before serving with carrot and mangetout vegetable fishes.

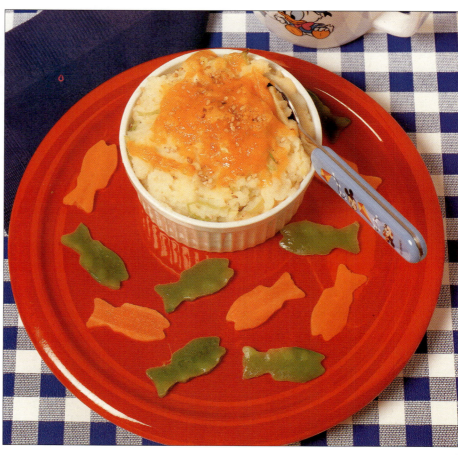

Cauliflower and Broccoli with Cheese

Serves 2

1 egg

75g/3oz cauliflower

75g/3oz broccoli

15g/½oz/1 tbsp margarine

15ml/1 tbsp plain (all-purpose) flour

150ml/¼ pint/⅔ cup milk

40g/1½oz/⅓ cup grated Red
  Leicester or mild cheese

½ tomato

salt and pepper (optional)

1 Put the egg in a small pan of cold water, bring to the boil and cook for about 10 minutes until the egg is hard-boiled.

2 Meanwhile, cut the cauliflower and broccoli into florets and thinly slice the broccoli stalks. Cook in a pan of boiling water for about 8 minutes, until just tender.

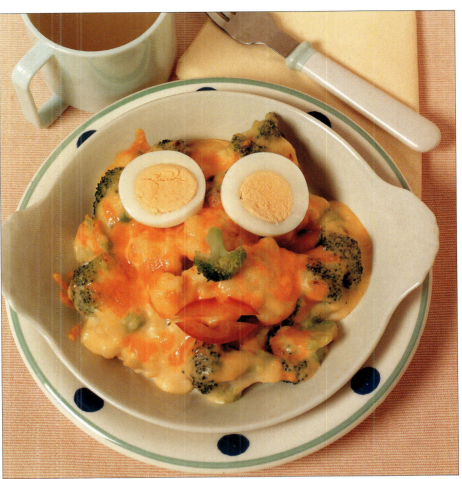

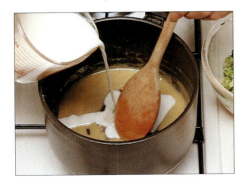

3 Drain the vegetables and dry the pan. Melt the margarine, stir in the flour, then gradually mix in the milk and bring to the boil, stirring until thickened and smooth.

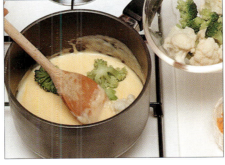

4 Stir two-thirds of the cheese into the sauce together with a little seasoning, if liked. Reserve two of the broccoli florets and stir the remaining vegetables into the sauce.

5 Divide the mixture between two heat-resistant shallow dishes and sprinkle with the remaining cheese.

6 Place under a hot grill (broiler) until golden brown and bubbling.

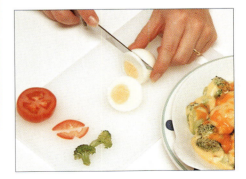

7 Make a face on each dish with broccoli florets for a nose, a halved tomato for a mouth and peeled and sliced hard-boiled egg for eyes. Cool slightly before serving.

TIP
Making a face or fun pattern can be just enough to tempt a fussy eater to try something new.

French Toast Butterflies

Serves 2

4 small broccoli florets
8 peas
1 small carrot
1 slice Red Leicester or mild cheese
2 slices ham
2 slices bread
1 egg
10ml/2 tsp milk
5ml/1 tsp vegetable oil
a little tomato ketchup

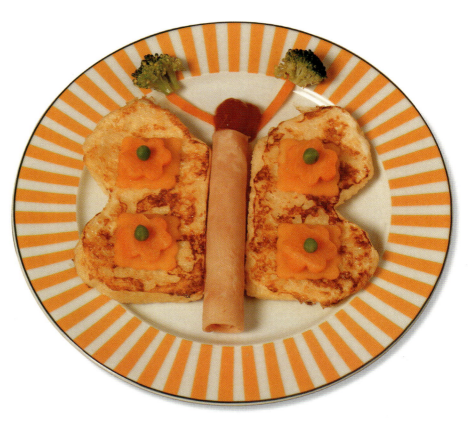

1 Cook the broccoli florets and the peas in a pan of boiling water for 5 minutes. Drain well.

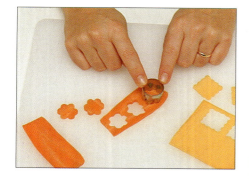

2 For each butterfly, cut four thin slices of carrot and cut into flower shapes with a petits four cutter. Cut out four small squares from the cheese.

3 Cut four thin strips from the rest of the carrot for antennae. Roll up each piece of ham and arrange in the middle of two serving plates, to make the two butterfly bodies.

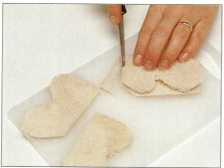

4 Cut butterfly wings from the bread, using a small knife.

TIP
Vary the ingredients for the butterfly decorations. Make a body from a grilled sausage if preferred.

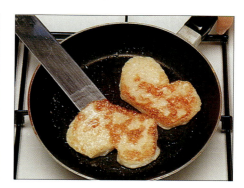

5 Beat together the egg and milk and dip the bread in the mixture to coat both sides thoroughly. Heat the oil in a medium-size frying pan and fry the bread until golden on both sides.

6 Assemble the butterfly, using the French toast for the wings and decorating with the carrot, cheese, broccoli and peas. Use a blob of ketchup for the head.

Pizza Clock

Serves 3–4

20cm/8in ready-made pizza base

45ml/3 tbsp tomato ketchup or pizza
  sauce

2 tomatoes

75g/3oz/¾ cup grated mild cheese

pinch of dried marjoram

1 green (bell) pepper

1 large carrot

1 thick slice ham

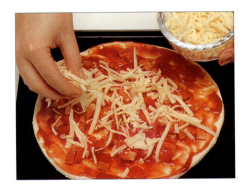

1 Preheat oven to 220°C/425°F/
Gas 7. Place the pizza base on a
baking sheet and spread with
ketchup or pizza sauce. Chop the
tomatoes and scatter over the pizza
with the cheese and marjoram.

2 Place directly on an oven shelf
and bake for 12 minutes, until
the cheese is bubbly. (Place a baking
tray on the shelf below the pizza to
catch any drips of cheese.)

TIP
If preferred, make a smaller version
of this using half a toasted muffin.
Top as above and grill (broil) until
the cheese melts. Add ham hands
and small pieces of carrot to mark
the numbers.

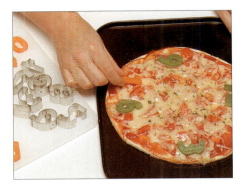

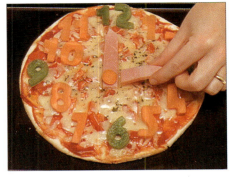

3 Meanwhile halve the pepper, cut
away the core and seeds and
stamp out the numbers 3, 6, 9 and 12
with small number cutters. Peel and
thinly cut the carrot lengthways and
stamp out the numbers 1, 2, 4, 5, 7,
8, 10 and 11. Arrange on the pizza to
form a clock face.

4 Cut out a carrot circle. Cut two
clock hands, each about 7.5cm/
3in long from the ham. Arrange on
the pizza with the circle of carrot.

5 Place the pizza clock on to a
serving plate and arrange the
numbers around the edge. Cool the
pizza clock slightly before cutting
into wedges and serving.

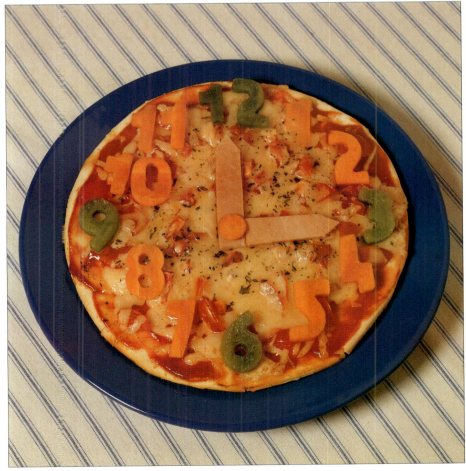

Pancakes

Serves 2–3

50g/2oz/⅓ cup plain (all-purpose)
  flour

1 egg

150ml/¼ pint/⅔ cup milk

15ml/1 tbsp vegetable oil

For the filling

1 banana

1 orange

2–3 scoops ice cream

a little maple syrup

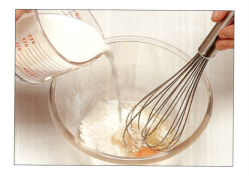

1 Sift the flour into a bowl, add the egg and gradually whisk in the milk to form a smooth batter. Whisk in 5ml/1 tsp of the oil.

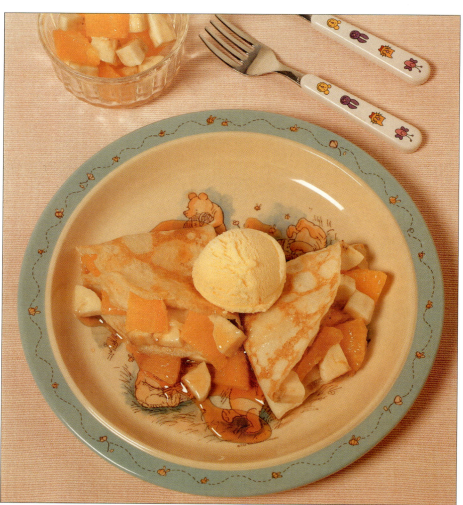

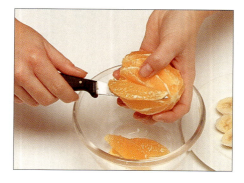

2 To make the filling, slice the banana thinly or in chunks. Cut the peel away from the orange with a serrated knife, then cut the orange into segments.

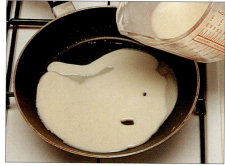

3 Heat a little of the remaining oil in a medium-size non-stick pan, pour off any excess oil and add 30ml/2 tbsp of the batter. Tilt the pan to evenly coat the base with the batter and cook for a couple of minutes, until the pancake is set and the underside is golden.

4 Loosen the edges with a knife, then toss the pancake or turn with a knife. Brown the other side and then slide out on to a plate. Fold in four and keep warm.

5 Cook the rest of the batter in the same way until you have made 6 pancakes. Place two on each plate.

6 Spoon a little fruit into each pancake and arrange on serving plates. Top with the remaining fruit and a scoop of ice cream, and pour over a little maple syrup. Serve at once.

Raspberry Sorbet

Makes: 900ml/1½ pints/3¾ cups

10ml/2 tsp powdered gelatine

600ml/1 pint/2½ cups water

225g/8oz/1¼ cups caster (superfine) sugar

675g/1½lb raspberries, hulled

grated rind and juice of ½ lemon

1 Put 30ml/2 tbsp water in a cup, sprinkle the gelatine over and set aside for a few minutes to soak.

2 Place the water and sugar in a pan and heat, stirring occasionally, until the sugar has completely dissolved.

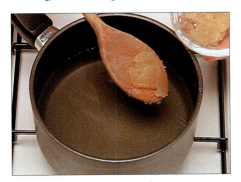

3 Bring to the boil and boil rapidly for 3 minutes. Remove from the heat, add the gelatine mixture to the syrup and stir until completely dissolved. Leave to cool.

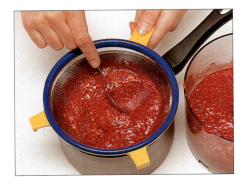

4 Liquidize or process the raspberries to a smooth purée, then press through a sieve (strainer) into the syrup. Stir in the lemon rind and juice.

5 Pour into a plastic tub and freeze for 6–7 hours, or until the mixture is half frozen.

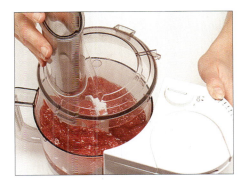

6 Beat the sorbet with a fork or transfer to a food processor and process until smooth. Return to the freezer and freeze until solid.

7 Remove the sorbet from the freezer 10 minutes before serving to soften slightly, then scoop into dishes with a melon baller or small teaspoon.

VARIATION
Summer Fruit Sorbet
Follow the recipe up to Step 3. Put a 500g/1¼lb pack of frozen summer fruits into a second pan. Add 60ml/ 4 tbsp water, cover and cook for 5 minutes until soft, then purée and sieve (strain), add to the syrup and continue as above.

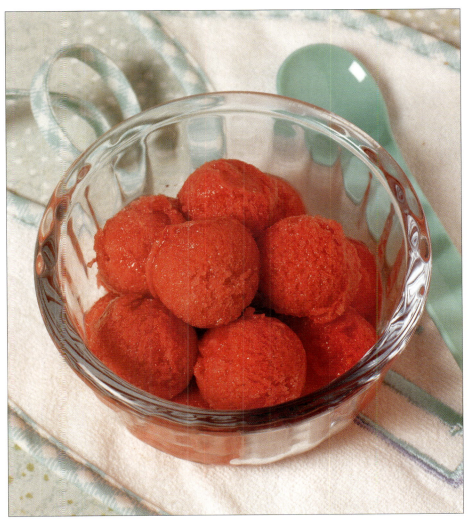

NUTRITIONAL INFORMATION

The nutritional analysis below is for the whole recipe.

p26 Vegetable Purée Energy 75Kcal/310kJ; Protein 2.6g; Carbohydrate 10.6g, of which sugars 10.1g; Fat 2.6g, of which saturates 1.6g; Cholesterol 8mg; Calcium 96mg; Fibre 2.4g; Sodium 51mg.

p27 Fruit Purées Energy 33Kcal/142kJ; Protein 0.7g; Carbohydrate 6.6g, of which sugars 6.6g; Fat 0.7g, of which saturates 0.4g; Cholesterol 2mg; Calcium 20mg; Fibre 1.1g; Sodium 8mg.

p32 Autumn Harvest Energy 420Kcal/1760kJ; Protein 15.4g; Carbohydrate 61.2g, of which sugars 35.7g; Fat 14g, of which saturates 8g; Cholesterol 42mg; Calcium 498mg; Fibre 11.4g; Sodium 199mg.

p33 Mixed Vegetable Platter Energy 412Kcal/1727kJ; Protein 19.3g; Carbohydrate 55.3g, of which sugars 28.5g; Fat 13.7g, of which saturates 8g; Cholesterol 42mg; Calcium 482mg; Fibre 8.6g; Sodium 190mg.

p34 Carrot, Lentil and Coriander Purée Energy 602Kcal/2531kJ; Protein 26.9g; Carbohydrate 97.5g, of which sugars 42.9g; Fat 13.9g, of which saturates 8.2g; Cholesterol 42mg; Calcium 478mg; Fibre 12.6g; Sodium 254mg.

p35 Red Pepper Risotto Energy 419Kcal/1744kJ; Protein 16g; Carbohydrate 60g, of which sugars 19.8g; Fat 12.6g, of which saturates 7.7g; Cholesterol 42mg; Calcium 409mg; Fibre 2.4g; Sodium 163mg.

p36 Parsnip and Broccoli Mix Energy 380Kcal/1590kJ; Protein 19g; Carbohydrate 43.7g, of which sugars 28g; Fat 15.2g, of which saturates 8.2g; Cholesterol 42mg; Calcium 511mg; Fibre 13.3g; Sodium 161mg.

p37 Turkey Stew with Carrots and Corn Energy 415Kcal/1756kJ; Protein 46.5g; Carbohydrate 49.2g, of which sugars 17.3g; Fat 4.9g, of which saturates 1.9g; Cholesterol 89mg; Calcium 96mg; Fibre 6.6g; Sodium 180mg.

p38 Chicken and Parsnip Purée Energy 544Kcal/2287kJ; Protein 43.8g; Carbohydrate 57.3g, of which sugars 33.5g; Fat 16.8g, of which saturates 8.6g; Cholesterol 123mg; Calcium 503mg; Fibre 16.1g; Sodium 233mg.

p39 Cock-a-Leekie Casserole Energy 523Kcal/2204kJ; Protein 43g; Carbohydrate 59.2g, of which sugars 18.2g; Fat 14g, of which saturates 8.2g; Cholesterol 123mg; Calcium 388mg; Fibre 3.9g; Sodium 229mg.

p40 Trout and Courgette Savoury Energy 561Kcal/2352kJ; Protein 41.6g; Carbohydrate 59.8g, of which sugars 18.9g; Fat 18.5g, of which saturates 8.6g; Cholesterol 119mg; Calcium 409mg; Fibre 4.3g; Sodium 214mg.

p41 Fisherman's Pie Energy 556Kcal/2338kJ; Protein 34.8g; Carbohydrate 76.2g, of which sugars 19g; Fat 14.2g, of which saturates 8.1g; Cholesterol 83mg; Calcium 389mg; Fibre 5.1g; Sodium 222mg.

p42 Apple Ambrosia Energy 308Kcal/1285kJ; Protein 11.8g; Carbohydrate 38.8g, of which sugars 19.5g; Fat 12.1g, of which saturates 7.5g; Cholesterol 42mg; Calcium 362mg; Fibre 1.1g; Sodium 130mg.

p43 Fruit Salad Purée Energy 142Kcal/604kJ; Protein 2.8g; Carbohydrate 33.8g, of which sugars 33.8g; Fat 0.4g, of which saturates 0g; Cholesterol 0mg; Calcium 35mg; Fibre 6.6g; Sodium 8mg.

p46 Sheperd's Pie Energy 487Kcal/2045kJ; Protein 29.4g; Carbohydrate 50.1g, of which sugars 15.2g; Fat 20.1g, of which saturates 8.4g; Cholesterol 69mg; Calcium 54mg; Fibre 5.3g; Sodium 379mg.

p47 Braised Beef and Carrots Energy 466Kcal/1959kJ; Protein 43.2g; Carbohydrate 50.7g, of which sugars 22.3g; Fat 11.3g, of which saturates 4.6g; Cholesterol 110mg; Calcium 91mg; Fibre 8g; Sodium 189mg.

p48 Lamb Hotpot Energy 365Kcal/1533kJ; Protein 26.8g; Carbohydrate 34.8g, of which sugars 16.7g; Fat 14.2g, of which saturates 6.3g; Cholesterol 87mg; Calcium 118mg; Fibre 7.2g; Sodium 159mg.

p49 Lamb and Lentil Savoury Energy 332Kcal/1397kJ; Protein 29.7g; Carbohydrate 24.4g, of which sugars 10.6g; Fat 13.6g, of which saturates 6g; Cholesterol 87mg; Calcium 97mg; Fibre 3.9g; Sodium 388mg.

p50 Country Pork and Runner Beans Energy 279Kcal/1174kJ; Protein 28.7g; Carbohydrate 30g, of which sugars 11.7g; Fat 5.7g, of which saturates 1.9g; Cholesterol 73mg; Calcium 71mg; Fibre 5.6g; Sodium 122mg.

p51 Pork and Apple Savoury Energy 410Kcal/1730kJ; Protein 42.5g; Carbohydrate 44.3g, of which sugars 16.9g; Fat 8.2g, of which saturates 2.6g; Cholesterol 110mg; Calcium 132mg; Fibre 6.4g; Sodium 170mg.

p52 Nursery Kedgeree Energy 625Kcal/2604kJ; Protein 39.2g; Carbohydrate 58.5g, of which sugars 16.3g; Fat 25.9g, of which saturates 12.1g; Cholesterol 494mg; Calcium 483mg; Fibre 1.2g; Sodium 223mg.

p53 Mediterranean Vegetables Energy 284Kcal/1202kJ; Protein 12.7g; Carbohydrate 54.5g, of which sugars 25.3g; Fat 3.1g, of which saturates 0.7g; Cholesterol 0mg; Calcium 89mg; Fibre 8.3g; Sodium 362mg.

p54 Pasta with Sauce Energy 608Kcal/2537kJ; Protein 30.8g; Carbohydrate 49.2g, of which sugars 27.6g; Fat 32g, of which saturates 20g; Cholesterol 98mg; Calcium 840mg; Fibre 6.4g; Sodium 545mg.

p55 Apple and Orange Fool Energy 219Kcal/924kJ; Protein 5.5g; Carbohydrate 37.6g, of which sugars 23.8g; Fat 6.1g, of which saturates 3.8g; Cholesterol 21mg; Calcium 188mg; Fibre 2.1g; Sodium 117mg.

p56 Orchard Fruit Dessert Energy 352Kcal/1492kJ; Protein 6.9g; Carbohydrate 71g, of which sugars 57.2g; Fat 6.3g, of which saturates 3.8g; Cholesterol 21mg; Calcium 233mg; Fibre 6.9g; Sodium 122mg.

p57 Peach Melba Dessert Energy 153Kcal/650kJ; Protein 7g; Carbohydrate 30.8g, of which sugars 30.8g; Fat 1.3g, of which saturates 0.6g; Cholesterol 2mg; Calcium 238mg; Fibre 1.7g; Sodium 98mg.

p66 Lamb Couscous Energy 631Kcal/2643kJ; Protein 40.6g; Carbohydrate 67g, of which sugars 39.3g; Fat 24.1g, of which saturates 9.6g; Cholesterol 133mg; Calcium 160mg; Fibre 6.6g; Sodium 227mg.

p67 Paprika Pork Energy 533Kcal/2248kJ; Protein 50.1g; Carbohydrate 60.2g, of which sugars 17.8g; Fat 11.9g, of which saturates 3.2g; Cholesterol 110mg; Calcium 132mg; Fibre 10.7g; Sodium 659mg.

p68 Chicken and Celery Supper Energy 331Kcal/1387kJ; Protein 39.5g; Carbohydrate 24.6g, of which sugars 22.1g; Fat 8.9g, of which saturates 2g; Cholesterol 184mg; Calcium 118mg; Fibre 7.3g; Sodium 285mg.

p69 Cauliflower and Broccoli with Cheese Energy 750Kcal/3127kJ; Protein 45.9g; Carbohydrate 50.2g, of which sugars 22.9g; Fat 39.9g, of which saturates 24.7g; Cholesterol 115mg; Calcium 1054mg; Fibre 9.4g; Sodium 720mg.

p70 Tagliatelle and Cheese with Broccoli and Ham Energy 668Kcal/2797kJ; Protein 42.9g; Carbohydrate 53.2g, of which sugars 17.4g; Fat 31.6g, of which saturates 19.3g; Cholesterol 120mg; Calcium 804mg; Fibre 4.4g; Sodium 1101mg.

p71 Baby Dhal Energy 305Kcal/1291kJ; Protein 18.1g; Carbohydrate 56.9g, of which sugars 16.6g; Fat 2g, of which saturates 0.4g; Cholesterol 0mg; Calcium 116mg; Fibre 8.8g; Sodium 59mg.

p72 Fish and Cheese Pie Energy 620Kcal/2595kJ; Protein 42.9g; Carbohydrate 49.2g, of which sugars 15.4g; Fat 27.9g, of which saturates 17.5g; Cholesterol 125mg; Calcium 701mg; Fibre 3.9g; Sodium 551mg.

p73 Fish Creole Energy 283Kcal/1185kJ; Protein 21.1g; Carbohydrate 46.4g, of which sugars 6.3g; Fat 1.2g, of which saturates 0.1g; Cholesterol 41mg; Calcium 43mg; Fibre 1.4g; Sodium 249mg.

p74 Chocolate Pots Energy 98Kcal/405kJ; Protein 5.8g; Carbohydrate 5.6g, of which sugars 5.5g; Fat 5.9g, of which saturates 2.8g; Cholesterol 106mg; Calcium 105mg; Fibre 0.1g; Sodium 77mg.

p75 Vanilla Custards Energy 94Kcal/392kJ; Protein 5.6g; Carbohydrate 5.5g, of which sugars 5.5g; Fat 5.7g, of which saturates 2.7g; Cholesterol 106mg; Calcium 104mg; Fibre 0g; Sodium 68mg.

p76 Marmite Bread Sticks Energy 15Kcal/63kJ; Protein 0.5g; Carbohydrate 2.4g, of which sugars 0.1g; Fat 0.4g, of which saturates 0.1g; Cholesterol 6mg; Calcium 4mg; Fibre 0.1g; Sodium 23mg.

p77 Bread Fingers with Egg Energy 14Kcal/58kJ; Protein 0.7g; Carbohydrate 1.8g, of which sugars 0.2g; Fat 0.5g, of which saturates 0.1g; Cholesterol 12mg; Calcium 8mg; Fibre 0.1g; Sodium 23mg.

p78 Cheese Straws Energy 41Kcal/172kJ; Protein 1.2g; Carbohydrate 3.3g, of which sugars 0.1g; Fat 2.6g, of which saturates 1.6g; Cholesterol 11mg; Calcium 27mg; Fibre 0.1g; Sodium 32mg.

p80 Mini Cup Cakes Energy 31Kcal/130kJ; Protein 0.4g; Carbohydrate 3.5g, of which sugars 2.1g; Fat 1.8g, of which saturates 0.1g; Cholesterol 7mg; Calcium 9mg; Fibre 0.1g; Sodium 25mg.

p81 Shortbread Shapes Energy 28Kcal/117kJ; Protein 0.3g; Carbohydrate 3.2g, of which sugars 0.9g; Fat 1.7g, of which saturates 1g; Cholesterol 4mg; Calcium 4mg; Fibre 0.1g; Sodium 12mg.

p86 Shepherd's Pie Energy 388Kcal/1617kJ; Protein 21.7g; Carbohydrate 28.7g, of which sugars 11.9g; Fat 21.5g, of which saturates 10.3g; Cholesterol 69mg; Calcium 69mg; Fibre 4.5g; Sodium 382mg.

p87 Lamb Stew Energy 152Kcal/635kJ; Protein 12.3g; Carbohydrate 7.5g, of which sugars 5g; Fat 8.4g, of which saturates 3.3g; Cholesterol 44mg; Calcium 29mg; Fibre 2.2g; Sodium 59mg.

p88 Fish and Cheese Pies Energy 300Kcal/1258kJ; Protein 19.3g; Carbohydrate 25.5g, of which sugars 6.5g; Fat 13.9g, of which saturates 7.8g; Cholesterol 59mg; Calcium 228mg; Fibre 1.6g; Sodium 246mg.

p89 Cauliflower and Broccoli with Cheese Energy 264Kcal/1101kJ; Protein 14.6g; Carbohydrate 11.9g, of which sugars 5.9g; Fat 17.6g, of which saturates 6.1g; Cholesterol 119mg; Calcium 293mg; Fibre 2.1g; Sodium 281mg.

p90 French Toast Butterflies Energy 243Kcal/1018kJ; Protein 17.2g; Carbohydrate 17g, of which sugars 3.9g; Fat 12g, of which saturates 5.2g; Cholesterol 127mg; Calcium 216mg; Fibre 2.4g; Sodium 615mg.

p91 Pizza Clock Energy 204Kcal/856kJ; Protein 10g; Carbohydrate 23.2g, of which sugars 9.3g; Fat 8.1g, of which saturates 4.3g; Cholesterol 25mg; Calcium 173mg; Fibre 2.2g; Sodium 547mg.

p92 Pancakes Energy 285Kcal/1194kJ; Protein 8.1g; Carbohydrate 33.3g, of which sugars 19.9g; Fat 14.2g, of which saturates 6.1g; Cholesterol 66mg; Calcium 163mg; Fibre 1.5g; Sodium 78mg.

p93 Raspberry Sorbet Energy 1055Kcal/4518kJ; Protein 10.6g; Carbohydrate 266.2g, of which sugars 266.2g; Fat 2g, of which saturates 0.7g; Cholesterol 0mg; Calcium 288mg; Fibre 16.9g; Sodium 34mg.

INDEX

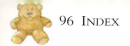